# Pediatric Bipolar Disorder
## A Handbook for Clinicians

# Pediatric Bipolar Disorder
## A Handbook for Clinicians

### Robert L Findling MD
Director of Child and Adolescent Psychiatry, Associate Professor of Psychiatry, University Hospitals of Cleveland, Case Western Reserve University, Cleveland, OH, USA

### Robert A Kowatch MD
Professor of Psychiatry and Pediatrics, Children's Hospital Medical Center of Cincinnati, University of Cincinnati Medical Center, Cincinnati, OH, USA

### Robert M Post MD
Chief, Biological Psychiatry Branch, National Institute of Mental Health, Bethesda, MD, USA

MARTIN DUNITZ

© 2003 Martin Dunitz Ltd, a member of the Taylor & Francis group

First published in the United Kingdom in 2003
by Martin Dunitz Ltd, Taylor & Francis Group plc, 11 New Fetter Lane, London
EC4P 4EE

Tel.: +44 (0) 20 7482 2202
Fax.: +44 (0) 20 7267 0159
E-mail: info@dunitz.co.uk
Website: http://www.dunitz.co.uk

Although every effort has been made to ensure that all owners of copyright
material have been acknowledged in this publication, we would be glad to
acknowledge in subsequent reprints or editions any omissions brought to our
attention.

A CIP record for this book is available from the British Library.

ISBN 1-84184-054-8

Distributed in the USA by
Fulfilment Center
Taylor & Francis
7625 Empire Drive
Florence, KY 41042, USA
Toll Free Tel.: +1 800 634 7064
E-mail: cserve@routledge_ny.com

Distributed in Canada by
Taylor & Francis
74 Rolark Drive
Scarborough, Ontario M1R 4G2, Canada
Toll Free Tel.: +1 877 226 2237
E-mail: tal_fran@istar.ca

Distributed in the rest of the world by
ITPS Limited
Cheriton House
North Way
Andover, Hampshire SP10 5BE, UK
Tel.:+44 (0)1264 332424
E-mail: reception@itps.co.uk

Composition by Wearset Ltd, Boldon, Tyne and Wear

Printed and bound in Great Britain by The Cromwell Press, Trowbridge

# Contents

# Contributors

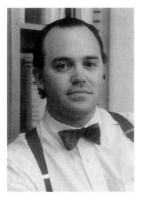

**Robert L Findling MD**

Dr Findling is the director of the Division of Child and Adolescent Psychiatry at Case Western Reserve University and University Hospitals of Cleveland. He is also an Associate Professor of Psychiatry and Pediatrics at Case Western Reserve University. Dr Findling earned his undergraduate degree at Johns Hopkins University and went to medical school at the Medical College of Virginia. Dr Findling did a joint residency–training program in Pediatrics, Psychiatry and Child & Adolescent Psychiatry at Mt Sinai Hospital in New York City. He is board certified in all three specialties.

Dr Findling's research endeavors have focused on pediatric psychopharmacology and psychotic disorders in the young. He has extensive experience in pharmacokinetic studies of psychotropic agents in pediatric patients. Dr Findling has been honored with numerous awards and has received international recognition as a clinical investigator. Dr Findling is currently the principal investigator of a Stanley Foundation Clinical Research Center that is examining novel interventions early in the course of juvenile bipolar illness. Dr Findling's current research is also supported in part from the NIH, the American Foundation for Suicide Prevention, the St Luke's Foundation of Cleveland, OH and the pharmaceutical industry.

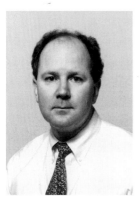

**Robert A Kowatch MD**

Dr Kowatch received his medical degree in 1980 and completed a residency in general psychiatry at the University of Pennsylvania Hospital in Philadelphia. He subsequently completed a fellowship in child and adolescent psychiatry at Hahnemann University in Philadelphia and is board certified in general psychiatry, child and adolescent psychiatry, and sleep disorders medicine.

In 1995, he was awarded an NIMH K-Award which he completed at the University of Texas Southwestern Medical Center at Dallas under the mentorship of Dr AJ Rush. In September 2000 he moved to Cincinnati where he is a Professor of Psychiatry and Pediatrics at the University of Cincinnati Medical Center and Children's Hospital Medical Center.

Dr Kowatch is active in several professional organizations including the American Academy of Child and Adolescent Psychiatry and the Society of Biological Psychiatry. He was chair of the Website/Information Technology Committee of American Academy of Child and Adolescent Psychiatry and is currently a member of the NIH Biobehavioral and Biobehavioral Processes 6 [BBBP-6] Study Section. He is on the editorial board of the *Journal of the American Academy of Child and Adolescent Psychiatry*, the *Journal of Child and Adolescent Psychopharmacology*, and *Current Psychiatry*.

His research interests are in the treatment of child and adolescent bipolar disorders and the neurobiology of these disorders. He is the principal coordinating investigator of a recently-funded, NIMH, multi-site, collaborative trial (1 RO1 MH63632-01) which is studying the efficacy of lithium and sodium divalproex in bipolar children and adolescents. He also is studying the neurobiology of affective lability of bipolar children and adolescents using functional MRI and various affective probes.

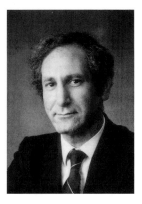

**Robert M Post MD**

Dr Post graduated from Yale University in 1964, the University of Pennsylvania School of Medicine in 1968, was a medical intern at the Einstein School of Medicine in 1969, and psychiatry resident at Massachusetts General Hospital for one year before joining the NIMH in 1970. After a clinical fellowship, he was promoted to Unit and Section Chief in the Biological Psychiatry Branch and has been Branch Chief for the past 18 years. Throughout his career he and his group have focused on better understanding and treating patients with refractory unipolar and bipolar illness.

Dr Post helped to pioneer the introduction of the anticonvulsant carbamazepine as a new therapeutic modality in lithium-refractory bipolar patients and has conducted studies of other anticonvulsants, including nimodipine, gabapentin, and lamotrigine, and most recently, non-convulsive brain stimulation with repetitive transcranial magnetic stimulation (rTMS). Exploration of some of the molecular mechanisms underlying behavioral sensitization, kindling, and tolerance phenomena in animal models has enabled him to reconceptualize illness recurrence and evolution at the level of cyclic alterations in gene expression.

Dr Post is the winner of major research awards from the Society of Biological Psychiatry, APA, ACNP, Anna Monika Foundation, NARSAD, and NDMDA, and is on the editorial boards of more than ten journals. He has published more than 800 scientific manuscripts, and was the founder and former head of the Stanley Foundation Bipolar Network.

# Preface

Bipolar disorders were once considered to be quite rare in children and adolescents. However, there is a growing body of scientific evidence to suggest that bipolar disorders are more prevalent than once believed. Moreover, over the past few years it also appears that the diagnosis of bipolar disorder has been considered at higher rates than in the past for an increasing number of pre-pubertal children who are suffering from a variety of disturbances of mood or behavior. These difficulties include 'mood swings', affective lability, irritability, aggression, impulsiveness, or agitation.

However, the diagnosis of bipolar disorder carries with it several implications that must not be taken lightly. In adults, bipolar disorders are considered to be chronic recurrent conditions. They require medication treatment. Adults with these bipolar disorders not only experience suffering from the direct effects on their mood, but these disorders can cause significant impairment in a person's vocational, intrafamilial, and interpersonal functioning. Therefore, assigning a diagnosis of a biopolar disorder to a child or teenager should be done carefully.

When a clinician is working with a youth for whom the diagnosis of bipolar is being considered, he or she is faced with a variety of difficulties both in the assessment process and the implementation of a treatment plan. Many symptoms of bipolar disorders are present in other psychiatric conditions and non-syndromal states in children and teenagers. Psychiatric co-morbidity is extremely common in children and adolescents, as well as adults, who suffer from bipolar disorders.

Besides difficulties with assessment, once a youngster is diagnosed with a bipolar disorder there are multiple vicissitudes associated with the treatment. Of course, the ultimate goal of treatment is symptom remission thus enabling children and teenagers with bipolar disorder to function in a developmentally appropriate fashion at home, with peers, and at school. Unfortunately, the need to treat these children and adolescents has outpaced the evidence-based scientific literature. Therefore, this volume represents a state-of-the-art overview of current and suggested practice, which hopefully will soon be supported by more definitive recommendations as the controlled trials literature accumulates.

The mainstays for the treatment of adult patients with bipolar disorder have been medications. The same is true for children and teenagers. However, the pharmacological management of juvenile bipolarity can often be a difficult undertaking for several reasons. Although many of the same agents appear to be useful in young people as in adults with bipolar disorders, at present there are no proven acute treatments or maintainence therapies for children or adolescents with this illness. Besides the paucity of well-controlled medication studies in this patient population that can be used to inform clinical practice, there are data to suggest that some of the compounds that are commonly used in adults may not be as well tolerated in children. In addition, several of the mood-stabilizing drugs have narrow therapeutic windows. Because of these considerations, it is often necessary that young people have blood samples obtained during the course of medication administration. Not surprisingly, phlebotomy is not generally well received by either young patients or their families.

Furthermore, when one considers pediatric psychopharmacological interventions, treating a patient with only a single agent has been generally considered optimal. However, there is a growing body of evidence to suggest that many youths with bipolar disorder require combination treatments. Unfortunately, it is not clearly defined which patients may be best suited for combination drug therapy. It is also unknown what medication combinations are most judiciously employed and implemented.

Besides the alleviation of target symptoms, the ultimate goal for treating any youngster with a psychiatric condition is enhancing the patients the ability to enjoy their lives, thrive at home, perform to their best potential in school, and develop rich and rewarding peer relationships. With these goals in mind, psychosocial interventions are often employed to complement the benefits that pharmacotherapy provides. Disappointingly there are few controlled studies of psychosocial interventions in this patient population.

However, despite the paucity of controlled data, much is known and a concencus is building about the assessment, neurobiology, and treatment of children and adolescents with bipolar disorder. Based on what is known, a rational approach to the assessment of these youngsters can be developed.

The demands of assessing and treating bipolar disorders in children and teenagers are many. Yet, with a careful and thoughtful approach to the evaluation and treatment of these patients, therapeutic successes can be achieved for most. The purpose of this book is to provide the reader with practical approaches to the evolving art and science of providing clinical care and treatment to children and adolescents with bipolar disorder.

# Acknowledgements

The authors would like to express thanks to the families who have participated in the research studies described in this book. It is a privilege to work with people and organizations that are committed to the betterment of children and teenagers who suffer from these conditions. We thank the Stanley Foundation for generously supporting clinically meaningful research in the field of pediatric bipolar disorder.

The artwork on the cover of this book is reproduced courtesy of NARSAD Artworks, a non-profit organization, which produces products featuring art by artists with mental illness. NARSAD Artwork's mission is to educate the public about mental illness and to change their view of those who suffer from these brain disorders. Its parent organization, the National Alliance for Research on Schizophrenia and Depression (NARSAD) is the largest public contributor-supported funder of research in these neurobiological disorders in the world.

We dedicate this volume to those parents and children who have struggled heroically with the ravages of childhood onset bipolar disorder at a time when guidance from physicians and the academic community has regretfully often lagged far behind their need. We hope this volume begins to help fill some of the gaps.

To my patients and their familes.

Robert Findling

To my family – Sharon, Ray and Sara – for putting up with me and my long work hours.

To my many teachers and mentors, including Drs A John Rush, Joe Digiacomo, Howard Baker, James Stinnett and VJ Maker, who provided me with the training and knowledge necessary to write this book.

Lastly, to the memory of Dr Warren Weinberg, who developed the original diagnostic criteria for bipolar disorders for children in 1978, and who helped thousands of children and adolescents with bipolar disorders recover and lead productive lives.

Robert Kowatch

To my patients, who have taught me so much and to my family – Susan, David, Laura and, most recently, Shannon – with whom I have been blessed.

Robert Post

# chapter 1

# Defining bipolar disorder

The term 'bipolar disorder' is often used as if the clinical manifestations that this term describes were a single entity. In fact bipolar disorder should be considered as a group of mood disorders. According to the current edition of the Diagnostic and Statistical Manual (DSM-IV), there are four different bipolar-related disorders. In the most recent iteration of the International Classification of Diseases (ICD-10), there are also four distinct types of bipolar disorders described. The various syndromes that constitute the group of bipolar disorders vary in their severity, duration of symptomatology, and prognosis. For these reasons, it is often best to consider bipolar disorder not as a single illness, but as a spectrum of conditions. However, for the sake of simplicity, the term bipolar disorder will be used throughout this book when referring to the group of syndromes that makes up the continuum of these affective disorders.

Since there is more than one type of bipolar disorder, it is not surprising that the clinical pictures of young patients with bipolar spectrum illnesses are remarkably diverse. However, there is another key explanation for the variability with which bipolar disorder may be manifest in the young. This comes from the fact that bipolar spectrum disorders are characterized by a variety of mood states that can exacerbate and remit over time.

# Mood states in bipolar disorder

When considering bipolar disorder it is essential to remember that these conditions are affective illnesses. Although significant behavioral difficulties can be present in children and adolescents with bipolar disorder, this is not a disruptive behavioral disorder. Therefore, a careful assessment of whether or not a youngster is experiencing the mood episodes that characterize these syndromes is essential.

It should also be remembered that bipolar disorder is a cyclic mood disorder. As such, a child's or adolescent's mood will fluctuate during the course of the illness. Therefore, as will be seen in subsequent chapters, it is paramount for the clinician not only to consider the mood state of the young patient that is present during the assessment period, but it is also vital to get a careful developmental and longitudinal history. Table 1.1 summarizes the variety of mood states that characterize bipolar spectrum disorders.

Kraepelin referred to bipolar disorder as 'manic-depressive insanity' due to the distinct mood episodes that characterize this condition. Besides 'manic' and 'major depressive' states, there are in fact several qualitatively different mood epochs that can occur during the course of a bipolar disorder. These affective periods can be characterized by whether they belong to the 'manic', 'depressive', 'euthymic', or 'mixed' group of mood episodes.

The mania-spectrum mood episodes consist of manic, hypomanic, and unspecified manic states. These mania-spectrum mood disturbances are characterized by an elevated, expansive, or irritable mood. To meet DSM-IV and ICD-10 criteria for a manic episode the mood state must be associated with moderate to severe dysfunction and must last at least one week.

What generally distinguishes hypomanic episodes from manic episodes is symptom severity. Hypomanic episodes are less severe. In addition, although patients can be in a hypomanic episode for weeks or months, the minimum duration criterion for a hypomanic episode is only 4 days. The final mania-spectrum mood episode is unspecified manic episodes that are of briefer duration than manic or hypomanic episodes, and are of variable symptom severity intensity. These unspeci-

Table 1.1  Different mood states in bipolar disorder

| Mood episode group | Subjective mood state(s) | Mood episode | Symptom severity | Minimum episode length |
|---|---|---|---|---|
| Mania | Elevated, expansive, irritable | Manic | Moderate–severe | ≥1 week |
| | | Hypomanic | Mild–moderate | ≥4 days |
| | | Unspecified manic | Mild–severe | <4 days |
| Depression | Depressed, irritable | Major depressive | Moderate–severe | ≥2 weeks |
| | | Dysthymic | Mild–moderate | 1 year |
| | | Unspecified depressive | Mild–Severe | Variable |
| Mixed | Depressed, elevated, expansive, irritable | Mixed | Moderate–severe | ≥1 week |
| | | Unspecified mixed | Moderate–severe | <1 week |
| Euthymic | Variable* | – | – | – |

*Although the patient's mood state is considered to be neutral, these youths may appear to be irritable, sad, anxious, or labile due to the presence of psychiatric co-morbidity or the presence of stressors.

fied manic episodes are characteristic of the most common form of pediatric bipolar disorder in DSM-IV, bipolar disorder not otherwise specified.

For a mood episode to be considered within the mania spectrum, other specific symptoms must also be manifest during the specific mood state. It is essential, however, to remember that the presence of these symptoms alone does not necessarily mean that these behaviors are truly symptoms of mania. These behaviors must either emerge or exacerbate to a significant degree during discrete epochs of abnormally elevated, expansive, or irritable mood episodes to be considered symptoms of mania/hypomania. In addition, it is also important that these symptoms, when present, are associated with a distinct change from prior functioning and are also present to a magnitude that is developmentally inappropriate.

For example, the degree of motoric activity present in a 6-year-old is typically greater than that seen in a 16-year-old. If a previously sedentary teenager develops significant difficulties with restlessness or hyperkinesis, although this level of activity might be considered normal for a 6-year-old, for the adolescent this might constitute the symptom of a mood disorder. Conversely, it is developmentally inappropriate for a pre-pubertal child to have an interest in sex to the same degree as a 17-year-old adolescent. Table 1.2 lists the different symptoms characteristic of bipolar mood states.

The syndromes that constitute the depression-related group of mood states include major depressive, dysthymic, and unspecified depressive episodes. Major depressive episodes are of moderate or greater severity and last for at least 2 weeks. In our experience, approximately half of the patients with bipolar I disorder have met symptom criteria for a major depressive episode at some point during the course of their illness. Dysthymia is associated with a lesser degree of dysfunction than major depression. However, unlike major depressive episodes which typically last for only a few months, dysthymia is a chronic condition in which the disturbance in mood is present for at least a year. The final syndrome in the depression-related group of mood states is the unspecified depressive episode. These are depressive episodes that do not meet symptom severity criteria or symptom duration criteria for either dysthymia or major depression.

Not surprisingly, the depression-related mood states are often characterized by a depressed mood. It should be noted, however, that depression-related disturbances in mood could also have irritability as the mood that is most prominently manifested. Also, there are additional symptoms that typically develop or become exacerbated during the

## Table 1.2  Symptoms of bipolar mood states

| *Symptoms of mania* | *Symptoms of depression* |
|---|---|
| **Behavior** | **Behavior** |
| • Agitation | • Agitation |
| • Decreased need for sleep | • Appetite decrease/weight |
| • Energy increase | decrease (insufficient for growth) |
| • Goal-directed activity increased | • Appetite increase/weight gain |
| • Rapid speech | (excessive) |
| • Restlessness | • Energy reduction |
| | • Excessive sleep |
| **Cognition** | • Insomnia |
| • Distractability | • Psychomotor retardation |
| • Flight of ideas | |
| • Grandiosity | **Cognition** |
| • Self-esteem increased | • Anhedonia |
| | • Confidence diminished |
| **Interpersonal** | • Concentration reduced |
| • High-risk pleasurable behavior | • Indecisiveness |
| • More talkative | • Morbid ideation |
| • Recklessness | |
| • Sexual behavior increased | **Emotional distress** |
| • Social disinhibition | • Emotional blunting |
| | • Guilt/self-reproach |
| | • Hopelessness |
| | • Self-esteem reduced |
| | • Suicidal plans, acts, ideation |
| | • Thoughts of death |

course of a depressive illness. Table 1.2 summarizes the symptoms that characterize the depression-related mood states.

Mixed states are those in which symptoms of mania and depression are both present. To meet DSM-IV criteria for a 'mixed episode' a patient must manifest symptoms of both a major depressive episode and a manic episode nearly every day during a 1-week period of time. Although it appears as if youngsters with bipolar disorder frequently present with simultaneously occurring symptoms of both depression and mania/hypomania (that is, with a 'mixed' presentation), the majority of young patients do not commonly experience 'mixed episodes' as they generally do not meet full symptom criteria for a major depressive disorder during epochs of mania.

It is paramount for the clinician who is evaluating a child or adolescent for whom a diagnosis of bipolar disorder is being considered to be familiar with how different mood states may be expressed. As young patients with bipolar spectrum disorders often appear quite irritable, knowing the specific manifestations of different mood states can facilitate an accurate diagnosis being made.

## Bipolar spectrum disorders

As noted above, there are four distinct bipolar disorders in the DSM-IV and four distinct bipolar disorders in the ICD-10. Presuming that the mood disturbance that is present is not due to a general medical condition or a substance-related event, a person meets ICD-10 diagnostic symptom criteria for bipolar affective disorder if the patient has had at least two episodes of hypomania or mania and has also experienced distinct periods of depressed mood. Conversely, in order to meet DSM-IV criteria for bipolar I disorder, a patient simply needs to have experienced a single episode of mania. Table 1.3 summarizes the different bipolar spectrum disorders listed in the DSM-IV and the ICD-10.

Bipolar II disorder, as defined by the DSM-IV, is characterized by the presence of at least one major depressive episode and at least one hypomanic episode in the absence of a manic or mixed episode. Other bipolar affective disorders, as defined by the ICD-10, include not only the symptom criteria for bipolar II disorder, but also recurrent manic episodes that occur without depression.

Cyclothymia is characterized in both the ICD-10 and DSM-IV by numerous distinct episodes of hypomanic symptoms and depressive symptoms. These symptoms are specifically delineated in the ICD-10, whereas they are not listed in detail in the DSM-IV. Whereas the DSM-IV precludes that a 2-month symptom-free period be present to meet diagnostic symptom criteria, this exclusionary criterion is not specified in the ICD-10. It should be noted that to meet the DSM-IV criteria for

## Table 1.3  Different bipolar spectrum disorders

| Diagnostic nosology | Specific disorder | Mania-related episode present | Depressed episode present |
|---|---|---|---|
| DSM-IV | Bipolar I | Manic, hypomanic, unspecified manic, mixed, or none | Major depressive, dysthymic, unspecified depressive, or none |
| | Bipolar II | Hypomanic, unspecified, or none | Major depressive, or none |
| | Cyclothymia | Hypomanic, unspecified, or none | Unspecified, or none |
| | Bipolar disorder not otherwise specified | Hypomanic, unspecified, or none | Major depressive, dysthymic, unspecified depressive, or none |
| ICD-10 | Bipolar affective disorder | Manic, hypomanic, unspecified manic, mixed, none | Major depressive, dysthymic, unspecified depressive, or none |
| | Other bipolar affective disorders | Manic, hypomanic, unspecified manic, mixed, or none | Major depressive, dysthymic, unspecified depressive, or none |
| | Bipolar affective disorder, unspecified | Manic, hypomanic, unspecified manic, mixed, none | Major depressive, dysthymic, unspecified depressive, or none |
| | Cyclothymia | Hypomanic, unspecified, or none | Unspecified, or none |

cyclothymia in adults, a 2-year duration of illness must be present. For children and adolescents, only a 1-year length of illness is necessary to meet the DSM-IV diagnostic symptom criteria for cyclothymia.

Bipolar affective disorder unspecified is used in the ICD-10 and bipolar disorder not otherwise specified (BP-NOS) is used in the DSM-IV when patients with significant, recurrent symptoms of mania, hypomania, and/or mixed states do not meet diagnostic symptom criteria for another bipolar spectrum disorder. As noted above, juveniles with a bipolar spectrum disorder most often suffer from BP-NOS. They have brief intense periods in which they have many of the symptoms of mania or hypomania. More often than not, their moods are irritable or dysphoric (and not elated) during these episodes.

When assessing young patients with bipolar affective disturbances, it is important for clinicians to be mindful of the spectral nature of bipolar disorder. This is because it appears that most youths with bipolar disorder do not suffer from the most severe expressions of bipolar illness. Rather, it seems as if BP-NOS and cyclothymia may be the most prevalent expressions of juvenile bipolarity.

## Psychotic features in bipolar disorders

Besides the mood states that characterize bipolar disorder, symptoms of psychosis may develop during the course of a bipolar illness. Psychosis can be present during periods of mania, depression, or during mixed episodes. In juveniles with bipolar disorder symptoms of psychosis are not consistently present throughout the course of the illness. When young patients with bipolar disorder do develop psychosis, these symptoms typically develop when those mood episodes are at their greatest severity. Delusions and auditory hallucinations appear to be the most common psychotic symptoms that occur in children and adolescents with bipolar disorder.

It appears as if the symptoms of psychosis that develop during these severe mood episodes are most often 'mood-congruent'. That is, when a young patient is experiencing an episode of mania, the symptoms of psychosis typically involve themes that are consistent with mood elevation. Thus, during periods of mania young people may develop delusions of grandeur, believe they have special abilities, and experience hallucinations expressing their sense of superiority or uniqueness. Conversely, during the depressed phases of illness youths with mood-congruent psychotic features may experience derogatory auditory hallucinations. They may also be preoccupied by delusions of guilt or worthlessness. Although 'mood-incongruent' psychotic features may occur in juveniles with bipolar disorder, they do not appear to occur as commonly as mood-congruent psychotic features.

## Course modifiers in bipolar disorders

The longitudinal course of bipolar disorder varies from patient to patient. To describe the longitudinal course of a child's or adult's illness, several 'course modifiers' are used. Patients are considered to be suffering from the 'rapid cycling' variant of bipolar disorder if they have experienced four or more distinct mood episodes within the previous 12 months. Delineating whether or not a patient suffers from bipolar disorder with rapid cycling may be an important consideration when evaluating a young person who is suffering from a bipolar illness. This is because in adults rapid cycling may be associated with differences in medication response that appears to be distinct when compared to patients without rapid cycling. Although it appears as if the rapid cycling variant of bipolar disorder in young people is relatively common, there are few data about whether or not rapid cycling affects medication response in juveniles. It should be noted that in adults rapid cycling appears to occur more commonly in females. Whether or not this is true in children and adolescents remains to be seen.

Another way in which the longitudinal course of a bipolar disorder can be characterized is by noting if a patient has experienced 'interepisode recovery'. A patient is noted to have experienced interepisode recovery if the patient has a complete remission of symptoms between the two most recent mood episodes. It appears as if interepisode recovery is relatively uncommon in juvenile bipolarity.

A seasonal pattern applicable to bipolar disorder depressive episodes is noted when there is a consistent seasonal relationship with onset of depressive episodes. In adults it appears as if higher rates of depressive episodes may occur in the fall.

## Epidemiology of pediatric bipolar disorders

At present it is generally accepted that the prevalence of bipolar I disorder in adults is approximately 1% with an equal male to female gender distribution. Furthermore, it appears as if an additional 1–3% of adults may suffer from one of the other bipolar spectrum conditions.

Bipolar disorder presents in a wide variety of ways in children and adolescents. This may be one of the reasons why there are so few epidemiological data regarding juvenile bipolarity when compared to what is known about adults with bipolar disorders. Unfortunately, there are almost no prevalence data regarding bipolar I disorder in children under the age of 13. However, it appears that approximately 1–3% of older adolescents suffer from a bipolar spectrum disorder. In addition, what data do exist suggest that bipolar I disorder is not the most common form of bipolar illness in teenagers. It appears as if BP-NOS is the most common form of bipolar illness during late adolescence. Although extensive epidemiological data are not available, it seems as if the male to female ratio for bipolar disorder for patients aged 5–17 years is approximately 2:1.

## Summary

'Bipolar disorder' is not one singular disorder. Bipolar illnesses are a spectrum of syndromes that vary in mood episode duration, symptom severity, and affective states. These mood episodes may also be complicated by the presence of psychosis. The longitudinal course of bipolar disorders can vary substantially between patients. For this reason, when faced with a youngster with affective disturbances (which are also associated with behavioral difficulties) it is important to consider the possibility that the patient may be suffering from one of a number of bipolar spectrum disorders. Just as important, it is vital for the clinician to be aware of the various ways in which children and adolescents with bipolar disorders may present themselves.

## Further reading

American Psychiatric Association (1994) *Diagnostic and Statistical Manual of Mental Disorders,* 4th edn. Washington, DC: American Psychiatric Association.

Carlson GA (1998) Mania and ADHD: co-morbidity or confusion. *J Affect Disord* **51**:177–87.

Emslie GJ, Rush AJ, Weinberg WA, Gullion CM, Rintelmann J, Hughes CW (1997) Recurrence of major depressive disorder in hospitalized children and adolescents. *J Am Acad Child Adolesc Psychiatry* **36**:785–92.

Findling RL, Calabrese JR (2000) Rapid-cycling bipolar disorder in children. *Am J Psychiatry* **157**:1526–7.

Findling RL, Gracious BL, McNamara NK, Calabrese JR (2000) The rationale, design, and progress of two novel maintenance treatment studies in pediatric bipolarity. *Acta Neuropsychiatrica* **12**:136–8.

Findling RL, Gracious BL, McNamara NK et al (2001) Rapid, continuous cycling and psychiatric co-morbidity in pediatric bipolar I disorder. *Bipolar Disord* **3**:202–10.

Geller B, Zimerman B, Williams M et al (2000) Diagnosis and characteristics of 93 cases of a prepubertal and early adolescent bipolar disorder phenotype by gender, puberty, and comorbid attention deficit hyperactivity disorder. *J Child Adolesc Psychopharmacol* **10**:157–64.

Kovacs M, Obrosky DS, Gatsonis C, Richards C (1997) First-episode major depressive and dysthymic disorder in childhood: clinical and sociodemographic factors in recovery. *J Am Acad Child Adolesc Psychiatry* **36**:777–84.

Kraepelin E (1921) *Manic-Depressive Insanity and Paranoia.* Edinburgh: Livingstone.

Lewinsohn PM, Klein DN, Seeley JR (1995) Bipolar disorders in a community sample of older adolescents: prevalence, phenomenology, comorbidity, and course. *J Am Acad Child Adolesc Psychiatry* **34**:454–63.

McElroy SL, Strakowski SM, West SA, Keck PE Jr., McConville BJ (1997) Phenomenology of adolescent and adult mania in hospitalized patients with bipolar disorder. *Am J Psychiatry* **154**:44–9.

Nottelmann E (2001) National Institute of Mental Health Research Roundtable on Prepubertal Bipolar Disorder. *J Am Acad Child Adolesc Psychiatry* **40**:871–8.

Silverstone T, Romans S, Hunt N, McPherson H (1995) Is there a seasonal pattern of relapse in bipolar affective disorders? A dual northern and southern hemisphere cohort study. *Br J Psychiatry* **167**:58–60.

Suppes T, Dennehy EB, Gibbons EW (2000) The longitudinal course of bipolar disorder. *J Clin Psychiatry* **61**(suppl 9): 23–30.

World Health Organization (1994) *International Classification of Disease and Related Disorders* (ICD-10). Geneva: World Health Organization.

# chapter 2

# Pediatric bipolarity – why now?

The topic of pediatric bipolar disorder has recently become the focus of a significant amount of attention. This has occurred both within the scientific community and amongst the general public. However, the observation that children and adolescents may suffer from bipolar illness or manic depression is not a new one. In fact, its occurrence in children has been recognized for over a century. What is even more interesting is that a recapitulation of many of the observations initially made about young patients with bipolar disorder, some of which are many decades old, can help elucidate why the topic of juvenile bipolarity is receiving so much attention today. Table 2.1 lists some of the historical concepts that contributed to the current theory of pediatric bipolar disorder.

## Historical overview

Mania has been recognized in young children since the 19th century. For example, there is a case report from the Liverpool Infirmary for Children that was published in 1884 that describes the clinical course of a manic episode in a 5-year-old girl. In that communication, the previously healthy child was noted to have developed 'acute mania' of approximately three weeks' duration. During this manic episode, the child was noted to have become 'wildly excited'. What is even more

Table 2.1 Historical concepts in juvenile bipolarity

*Core historical concepts*
- There may be a childhood variant of bipolar disorder
- Juvenile bipolarity may be difficult to identify
- Symptom overlap exists with other psychiatric disorders
  Psychotic
  Depressive
  Anxiety
  Disruptive behavioral disorders

- Co-morbidity with other psychiatric disorders is possible
- Bipolar disorder in childhood is rare
- Irritability or mixed states characterize manic episodes

*Clinical relevance*
- If a childhood-specific expression of bipolar disorder exists, it has yet to be definitively characterized. This may be due to difficulties with the juvenile-onset variant and psychiatric co-morbidities
- Symptoms of psychosis, depression, anxiety, and disruptive behavior disorders occur in youths with a bipolar spectrum disorder
- Patients with juvenile bipolar disorders need to have the possibility of other co-morbid diagnoses considered
- Bipolar disorder in childhood is often not considered in the differential diagnosis
- Elation does not generally characterize manic episodes

interesting is that it appears that this child seems to have experienced a depressive episode prior to the onset of mania. During this episode of depression, the young girl lost weight, developed somatic complaints, and was 'inclined to sit about'.

Kraepelin suggested that bipolar disorder, albeit uncommon in children, was relatively common during the second half of the second decade of life. Kraepelin observed that by the age of 20 approximately 19% of patients had developed their first episode of 'manic-depressive insanity'. He also noted that the overwhelming majority of patients who developed their first episode of manic depression during their adolescence did so between the ages of 15 and 20. Approximately 16% of all patients experienced their first 'attack' of manic-depressive insanity between the ages of 15 and 20 years. Only about 3% of patients developed bipolar illness prior to the age of 15. Moreover, Kraepelin noted that less than 1% of patients with this condition experienced their first episode during their first 10 years of life.

A subsequent report that supported the contention that bipolar disorder was uncommon in children was published in the 1930s. In a series of 10 patients between the ages of 10 and 15 years, Kasanin not only noted that bipolar disorder was uncommon in children, but also considered several other themes pertaining to juvenile bipolarity. All of these concepts remain pertinent today, many decades after these observations were initially published. One theme was that it might be difficult to distinguish hypomanic episodes in the young as children are typically more motorically active than adults. Another concept considered by Kasanin was making the distinction between what today might be considered attention-deficit/hyperactivity disorder (ADHD) and juvenile bipolarity. Kasanin noted that because some children are chronically restless, what distinguished these chronically restless patients from those with juvenile mania was 'well-defined periods of elation or depression'. Finally, Kasanin noted that youths with bipolar disorder were at risk for being misdiagnosed as suffering from schizophrenia.

The next case series that described a sizable number of pediatric patients with bipolarity was published in the 1950s. In that report, in which 18 children were described, Campbell noted that an earlier age at onset of cyclothymia or manic depression was associated with a significant propensity for a family history of similar conditions. This is an important observation of clinical relevance because it suggests that a careful family history is important when considering the diagnosis of bipolar spectrum disorders in children and adolescents. Campbell also noted that youngsters with bipolar spectrum disorders are often misdiagnosed. Initial diagnoses frequently given to these patients included 'psychoneurosis' or schizophrenia. In addition, these youths could have disruptive behaviors and be considered as 'problem children'. Because young people with bipolar disorders can appear anxious, disruptive, or psychotic, correctly diagnosing whether or not a youth suffers from a bipolar disorder can be a difficult task. In fact, concerns about how to most accurately diagnose bipolar disorder in juveniles with a variety of different symptoms persist even today.

The first attempt to develop a set of diagnostic symptom criteria for childhood mania was published by Weinberg and Brumback in 1976. These authors emphasized several points. They noted that during manic episodes in children, high rates of depressive symptomatology were also present. In addition, they recognized that irritability was prominent during manic episodes. It was also noted that episodic hyperactivity was different from 'hyperactive child syndrome' because the latter was characterized by chronic, persistent over-activity. As a heuristic example, they also described a child whose chronic hyperactivity was well controlled with psychostimulants, but had spontaneous episodes of superimposed mood disturbances.

The possibility of there being a childhood variant of bipolar disorder was also noted by Davis (1979) who suggested that 'affective storms' are present in children with bipolar disorder. These 'storms' were described as periods characterized by brief, transient episodes of affective dysregulation. During these episodes, temper outbursts occurred and the affected children typically overreacted to an external precipitant or stressor. Aggressive behavior, hyperactivity, and violent behavior were also noted as possible characteristics of these outbursts. It should be noted that Davis also asserted that a chronic course, an absence of psychotic thinking, and a positive family history of a mood disorder were also necessary prior to making this diagnosis.

In summary, during the first decades in which juvenile bipolarity was described in the medical literature, several historical themes have recurred. One theme is that pediatric bipolar disorder may be confused with schizophrenia. A recent survey of 93 youths with juvenile-onset bipolar disorder suggested that more than half of patients with a bipolar disorder had a psychotic symptom. Although it appears that the syndrome of psychosis per se may not be this common in juvenile bipolar disorder, it is clear that patients with psychosis and bipolar illnesses may be diagnosed with schizophrenia.

Besides being misdiagnosed with schizophrenia, another theme that has been noted for decades is that youths with bipolar disorder can be quite disruptive or appear anxious. Therefore, these youths may receive other inaccurate diagnoses as well. What confounds this matter further is the notion raised by Weinberg and Brumback that apparent co-morbidity with other psychiatric conditions can also occur in young people with bipolar disorder.

Another group of interrelated themes revolve around the prevalence of juvenile bipolarity. Kraepelin, Kasanin, and others have historically asserted that childhood bipolar disorder is a rare phenomenon. There are no epidemiological data about the prevalence of bipolar disorder during childhood. To this day, others have also suggested that this condition is quite uncommon in the young. However, since symptoms of bipolar disorder may overlap with other forms of psychopathology, it is possible, as suggested by Davis (1979), that a childhood variant of bipolar disorder may not be readily recognized. If this is the case, it is also possible that childhood bipolar disorder may not be so rare after all.

## Current interest in pediatric bipolarity

There are several reasons why interest in pediatric bipolarity has become intense. One is the assertion that bipolar disorder during childhood and adolescence is not as rare as once presumed. As noted above, the assertion that bipolar disorder was relatively uncommon was typically agreed upon by consensus of opinion. However, recent epidemiological data suggest that although bipolar I disorder may not be common among late adolescents, less severe bipolar spectrum disorders might be reasonably common with approximately 1% of late adolescents suffering from these conditions. In addition, many adults with bipolar illness note that the symptoms of their illness began during childhood. Moreover, there is evidence to suggest that the reason more pediatric patients are suffering from bipolar illness during the first two decades of life is that an earlier age at onset of this illness is occurring within each subsequent generations in those with a family history of bipolar disorder.

If juvenile bipolar disorder is not as rare as once presumed, it is possible that young people with bipolar spectrum disorders are not being accurately diagnosed and not being effectively treated. This has led to some concerns that bipolar disorder may go under-diagnosed in some patients. In summary, more recent evidence suggests that bipolar spectrum disorders may develop in children and adolescents more frequently than previously presumed. However, when bipolar disorder does occur in young people, the more typical 'adult' illnesses of bipolar I disorder and bipolar II disorder are not as frequently seen in this population as bipolar disorder not otherwise specified and cyclothymia. Therefore, the more common expressions of bipolar disorders during childhood and adolescence are more subtle than those seen in adults. For this reason, the manifestations of bipolar disorder may be more difficult to detect and accurately diagnose. Unfortunately, there are substantial risks associated with inappropriately assigning a diagnosis of bipolar disorder to someone without the condition as well as eschewing the diagnosis of bipolar disorder in someone who does. These will be considered in detail in subsequent chapters.

## Summary

A review of how pediatric bipolarity has been conceptualized over the decades as well as a consideration of why juvenile bipolar disorder has recently received more attention than ever is important for several reasons. A significant number of young inpatients and outpatients seen in mental health settings have been reported to suffer from bipolar disorders. Therefore, there is a significantly large group of youngsters in mental health settings who deserve treatment. However, it has also been clear over the decades that accurately making a diagnosis of bipolar disorder in a young person is not an easy undertaking. Because these youths may be psychotic, disruptive, depressed, or anxious, they may be easily misdiagnosed with any number of other psychiatric conditions.

Probably of greater importance is the appreciation that most youths with bipolar spectrum disorders do not generally meet diagnostic symptom criteria for bipolar I disorder or bipolar II disorder. These youths generally have more subtle expressions of this condition, most of whom do not appear to present for mental health treatment. As these youths have more modest expressions of bipolar illness, they appear to be even more difficult to diagnose than those children and teenagers with more 'full' expressions of bipolar disorder.

Despite the problems associated with accurately diagnosing bipolar disorders in a young person, the stakes associated with an accurate diagnosis are quite high. Over-diagnosis can be associated with chronic medication treatment, stigmatization, and unnecessary psychological sequelae. Under-diagnosis can lead to needless human suffering. In addition, delays in receiving care may make the condition less responsive to treatment at a later time.

What further complicates the issue is the concern that youths who do suffer from the most severe expression of bipolar disorder may suffer from a juvenile variant of the illness. As this variant has not been definitively characterized, practitioners have become concerned about who may and may not be suffering from this juvenile bipolar variant. Unfortunately, there is no laboratory test, neuroimaging study, or neuropsychological probe that can definitively either confirm or refute the diagnosis of a bipolar spectrum disorder in a child or a teenager.

A historical review reveals that bipolar disorder changes its expression across months and years. By the time many youths present for care, they have often been quite symptomatic for years. They have often been misdiagnosed. It is possible that by focusing on the early expressions and the natural history of juvenile bipolar disorder, clinicians may find it easier to make an accurate diagnosis in a child or adolescent who presents for clinical care.

## Further reading

Campbell JD (1952) Manic depressive psychosis in children. Report of 18 cases. *J Nerv Ment Dis* **116**:424–39.

Carlson GA, Fennig S, Bromet EJ (1994) The confusions between bipolar disorder and schizophrenia in youth: where does it stand in the 1990s? *J Am Acad Child Adolesc Psychiatry* **33**:453–60.

Carlson GA, Strober M (1978) Manic-depressive illness in early adolescence. A study of clinical and diagnostic characteristics in six cases. *J Am Acad Child Psychiatry* **17**:138–53.

Davis RE (1979) Manic-depressive variant syndrome of childhood: a preliminary report. *Am J Psychiatry* **136**:702–6.

Geller B, Zimerman B, Williams M et al (2000) Diagnostic characteristics of 93 cases of prepubertal and early adolescent bipolar disorder phenotype by gender, puberty, and comorbid attention deficit hyperactivity disorder. *J Child Adolesc Psychopharmacol* **10**:157–64.

Greves EH (1884) Acute mania in a child of five years; recovery; remarks. *Lancet* **ii**:824–6.

Kasanin J (1931) The affective psychoses in children. *Am J Psychiatry* **10**:897–926.

Kraepelin E (1921) *Manic-Depressive Insanity and Paranoia*. Edinburgh: Livingstone.

Lewinsohn PM, Klein DN, Seeley JR (1995) Bipolar disorders in a community sample of older adolescents: prevalence, phenomenology, comorbidity, and course. *J Am Acad Child Adolesc Psychiatry* **34**:454–63.

Post RM, Weiss SRB, Leverich GS, George MS, Frye M, Ketter TA (1996) Developmental psychobiology of cyclic affective illness: implications for early therapeutic intervention. *Dev Psychopathol* **8**:273–305.

Weinberg WA, Brumback RA (1976) Mania in childhood. Case studies and literature review. *Am J Dis Child* **130**:380–5.

# chapter 3

# The development of bipolar disorders

The symptoms of depression and mania that occur in young people afflicted with any of the bipolar disorders can at times be of relatively modest intensity whereas at other times they can be quite pronounced. Because these disorders constitute a spectrum of illnesses, youths with bipolar disorders can be impaired to a variety of different degrees. Dysfunction can occur in several different domains.

Patients with bipolar disorders may have difficulties with academic achievement and deportment in school. Similarly, youths with bipolar disorders (and their families) can experience substantial distress and unhappiness due to intrafamilial conflict. Peer relationships can also be adversely affected by this illness. However, the degrees of impairment experienced by patients with bipolar spectrum disorders do not appear equal across these conditions. At present it appears as if young patients with either bipolar I or bipolar II disorder are generally more impaired than youths with bipolar disorder not otherwise specified (BP-NOS) or cyclothymia.

Bipolar disorders can be considered as a group of *progressive* illnesses. It has been shown that the mood episodes that characterize these conditions can become more severe and more prolonged over time. Therefore, patients may initially experience relatively brief and more modest affective episodes earlier in the course of their illness. Because of the brevity and modest severity of these first mood states, patients may initially meet diagnostic symptom criteria for either cyclothymia or bipolar

Table 3.1  Evidence that bipolar disorder may be a progressive illness over time

| Characteristic | Change with time |
| --- | --- |
| Severity | Modest episodes become more profound |
| Frequency | Interepisode periods become abbreviated; rate of cycling becomes more rapid |
| Autonomy | Cycles initially occur after a stressor; they subsequently develop spontaneously |
| Tolerance | Previously effective therapies may no longer work |
| Refractoriness | Discontinuation of a previously effective medication can lead to relapses that are no longer responsive to the previous agent |
| Ultradian fluctuations | Extreme rapidity of cycles can occur in later stages, but may also be characteristic of the earliest forms |
| Polypharmacy | Later in the course of illness, affective episodes may not respond to a single drug |

disorder NOS. These patients may eventually meet diagnostic symptom criteria for either bipolar I or bipolar II disorder. For many patients with bipolar I or bipolar II disorder, their illness can be conceptualized as the end result of either cyclothymia or bipolar disorder NOS. Table 3.1 summarizes the information regarding bipolar disorder as a progressive illness.

Besides mood episode length and severity, there are other ways in which bipolar disorders appear to change over time. For example, there are data from reports in adults that have noted that the rates of cycling between mood states may increase over time. As a result of this phenomenon, two distinct events occur. First, fluctuations between mood states may occur more rapidly. Second, it also seems that the amount of time that patients spend between mood states (e.g. euthymic) also becomes reduced.

In addition, although the mood states associated with these conditions are often precipitated by stressors early in the course of the illness, there are data to support the assertion that cycling becomes more autonomous over time. That is, early in the course of the illness the mood cycles that occur typically develop after an external trigger has precipitated them. However, later on these affective episodes eventually begin to develop spontaneously.

As discussed in Chapters 7 and 8, pharmacotherapy is the mainstay of treatment for bipolar disorders. It should be noted that there are data to suggest that a patient's response to medication therapy may change over time. For example, affective episodes may become more treatment resistant to previously effective drugs with each new cycle that a patient experiences. In addition, it appears as if, over time, patients who were initially responsive to treatment with only one medication may eventually only receive optimal benefit from treatment with two or more agents.

Based on the available data, it is possible that bipolar disorders may be most amenable to treatment during the initial stages of the illness. With this in mind, the rationale for intervention early in the course of a bipolar spectrum disorder becomes evident. As many patients with bipolar illness note that the symptoms of their illness were present, but undiagnosed, during childhood and adolescence, it may be quite important to be able to identify these patients during the pre-adult years. There are data from several lines of research to suggest that adult patients with bipolar I disorders may indeed have a variety of mood and behavioral symptoms during childhood and adolescence that may serve as early warning signs for the subsequent development of bipolar disorder. If these early symptoms were better appreciated, particularly in genetically at-risk children and adolescents, it is possible that specific *preventative* interventions could be developed for these patients.

One of the methods that have been used to examine and describe the antecedent symptoms of bipolar disorder has been a retrospective approach in afflicted adults. In this form of study, childhood psychiatric histories of adults with bipolar disorder are examined. Another line of investigation is that of high-risk studies. As heredity is a known risk factor for developing bipolar disorder, youths who are the offspring of a parent with bipolar illness are at genetically higher risk of developing the condition. Studies have been performed that have specifically examined the psychological and behavioral status of this at-risk group. Finally, there has been some epidemiological research that has been performed in adolescents that has considered the prevalence of bipolar disorders in this age group. What follows is a selected review regarding the data that are available from each of these lines of research.

## Retrospective research

There has been surprisingly little methodologically rigorous research that has retrospectively studied the childhood antecedents of bipolar disorder in adults who suffer from this condition. However, in one study, 100 adults with a variety of mood disorders were examined in a retrospective chart review. In that study it was found that almost one in three of these patients were brought for psychiatric assessment during their childhood (Manzano and Salvador, 1993). Interestingly enough, depression, irritability, and mood elevation were not the reasons for referral during childhood. Hyperactivity, educational difficulties, and anxiety were the chief concerns that led these patients' guardians to seek psychiatric consultation for their children.

The results of this study may be interpreted to suggest that anxiety and behavioral difficulties are potentially prodromal symptoms of bipolar disorder in the young. Another possibility is that subtle, underappreciated mood symptoms are present in youths who eventually develop bipolar disorder. It may be just that these more modest affective states are difficult to diagnose accurately. Therefore, the more readily identifiable symptoms of anxiety, agitation, and academic underachievement may be the manifestations of bipolar disorder that are most easily appreciated by both parents and clinicians.

Retrospective research has also highlighted that many patients with bipolar disorder develop symptoms of their illness during childhood and adolescence. The National Depressive and Manic-Depressive Association is a support and advocacy group, located in the United States, for patients with mood disorders and their families. In a retrospective survey of this group's members with bipolar illness, more than half of the respondents noted that they experienced the first symptoms of their condition during the pre-adult years (Lish et al 1994). Some 31% noted that they had initial manifestations of bipolar disorder during childhood. Another 28% reported that they first experienced symptoms of their affective illness during adolescence. Delays in looking for treatment were prevalent: 80% of respondents with childhood- or adolescent-onset bipolar illness had a greater than one year period of delay prior to seeking treatment. In addition, based on the results of this survey, it appeared that illness onset during the pre-adult years was associated with a family history of bipolar illness. Furthermore, this study also described that frequently recurring mood symptomatology in the respondents was associated with an early age at onset.

Both of these studies highlight the need for accurate, prompt diagnosis for patients with early-onset bipolar disorder. The findings from the National Depressive and Manic-Depressive Association retrospective survey point out the need to develop means by which early identification can occur and preventative interventions may be implemented for youths at genetically high risk of developing this condition.

## High-risk studies in children and teenagers

There has been more research done in children and adolescents who are the offspring of a parent with bipolar disorder, and are therefore at genetically high risk of developing the illness. One of the largest studies involved 68 at-risk youths between the ages of 6 and 24 years who were brought for clinical care (Akiskal et al 1985). These subjects were either the offspring or a younger sibling of a patient with bipolar disorder. The authors noted that depression, dysthymia, and cyclothymia were the most common diagnoses for these patients. These data highlight that the more severe forms of bipolar disorder were not the most common diagnoses in this population, but that depression and more subtle forms of affective symptoms were most prevalent.

Another study compared the psychological status of teenagers who were the offspring of a parent with bipolar disorder to a group of adolescents whose parents were psychiatric patients but did not have mood disorders (Klein et al 1985). The authors noted that the youths at genetically high risk of bipolar disorders had higher rates of psychopathology and higher rates of mood disorders than the comparison group. Moreover, although none of the high-risk offspring met symptom criteria for bipolar I disorder, the most common psychiatric disorder seen in this group was cyclothymia. The results of this study again highlight the need to more readily consider and accurately identify less severe forms of bipolar illness in genetically at-risk young people.

In another study of child and adolescent offspring of bipolar parents, high rates of psychopathology were noted. Depressive, anxious, and disruptive behavior disorders were commonly observed (Grigoroiu-Serbănescu et al 1989). Other, smaller studies of genetically at-risk children have also highlighted the high rates of depressive illnesses and disruptive behavior disorders in this population.

The finding that disruptive behavior disorders are common in offspring of parents with bipolar disorder has been noted in several studies. For example, a recent survey of the psychopathology of 60 youths who were the offspring of one or two parents with bipolar disorder and who were also between the ages of 6 and 18 years has recently been published (Chang et al 2000). In this study, the authors noted that approximately half of their subjects had a diagnosable psychiatric illness. Interestingly enough, the most common diagnosis seen in this cohort was attention-deficit hyperactivity disorder (ADHD). In fact, ADHD was seen almost twice as often as either a bipolar spectrum disorder or a depressive spectrum illness. It was also observed that an earlier age at onset of the illness for the affected parent(s) or a parental history of ADHD was associated with an increased risk of their children developing a bipolar disorder.

Others have also suggested that the presence of disruptive behavior disorders in youths who are the children of bipolar parents may have particular significance. In a large study in which the offspring of parents with bipolar disorder were compared to offspring of other psychiatric patients, high rates of attention and behavior problems during childhood were noted (Carlson and Weintraub 1993). However, the authors found that affective symptomatology during the early adult years was associated with attention and behavior problems during childhood only in the bipolar at-risk group but not the other cohort of offspring of psychiatric patients.

There are also data to suggest that infants and toddlers at genetically high risk of bipolar disorder may have difficulties as well. Difficulties with affective regulation and social development have been reported in a small study of 7 infants during the second year of life (Gaensbauer et al 1984). A follow-up of these children at the age of 6 noted they had high rates of symptoms of depression, anxiety, and disruptive behaviors (Zahn-Waxler et al 1988).

In summary, the data show that children and adolescents who have at least one parent with bipolar disorder are at high risk for having psychiatric symptomatology during childhood or adolescence. Mood and disruptive behavior disorders appear to be the most common. It appears the most readily identified mood disorders in these young people are depressive spectrum illnesses and cyclothymia. Bipolar I and bipolar II disorder seem to be less common. Unfortunately, accurate and early diagnosis does not seem to occur readily in this group of young people. Means of addressing this very important issue should be a topic for future research.

## Epidemiological study

Unfortunately, there are few data available about the incidence or prevalence of bipolar disorder in young people. What information is available suggests that the prevalence of bipolar spectrum disorders is approximately 1% during late adolescence. Moreover, the most common forms of bipolar illness during this period of life may be bipolar II disorder or cyclothymia. Only approximately one-half of patients identified with bipolar spectrum disorders in this study had received treatment (Lewinsohn et al 1995).

## Summary

Based on the available data from several avenues of research in children and adolescents, it appears that the longitudinal course of bipolar disorder is indeed a progressive one. Early in the course of the condition, periods in which manic symptoms occur appear to be more modest and less protracted than subsequently seen. However, it also appears that symptoms of anxiety and depression are common initial manifestations of bipolar illness. Moreover, disruptive behaviors are also common in at-risk youths. Whether these behavioral difficulties are indeed a true prodrome of this condition or an epiphenomenon remain to be seen. Table 3.2 lists key developmental concepts in bipolar illness.

Because of the apparent progressive nature of these conditions, intervention during the earliest phases may be ideal. Based on the available information, it appears that genetically at-risk youths with bipolar disorder BP-NOS or cyclothymia may be a reasonable group to consider for treatment studies. Unfortunately, there are almost no treatment data for this population. What does exist suggests that pharmacological agents that are effective for adults with bipolar disorders are effective treatments for this group of patients. However, it is important to remember that not all youngsters who report manic symptoms necessarily have a bipolar disorder. Future studies should focus on means by which accur-

Table 3.2 Key developmental concepts in bipolarity

Subsyndromal symptoms often develop during childhood and adolescence

Misdiagnosis seems commonplace; errors of omission seem most common

Treatment delays often occur

Depression, dysthymia, and cyclothymia may be initial manifestations; more severe forms of bipolarity may subsequently develop

Anxiety and disruptive behaviors may antecede the development of mood episodes

ate assessment and safe effective treatment can be given to young people earlier in the course of a bipolar illness.

There are some data to suggest that a parent-report version of the General Behavior Inventory (GBI) may be promising as an instrument to identify accurately young patients with mood disorders (including those with more modest forms of bipolar illness). Whether or not this is truly the case should be a topic for future research.

## Further Reading

Akiskal HS, Downs J, Jordan P, Watson S, Daugherty D, Pruitt DB (1985) Affective disorders in referred children and younger siblings of manic-depressives. Mode of onset and prospective course. *Arch Gen Psychiatry* **42**:996–1003.

Carlson GA, Kashani JH (1988) Manic symptoms in a non-referred adolescent population. *J Affect Disord* **15**:219–26.

Carlson GA, Weintraub S (1993) Childhood behavior problems and bipolar disorder – relationship or coincidence? *J Affect Disord* **28**:143–53.

Chang KD, Steiner H, Ketter TA (2000) Psychiatric phenomenology of child and adolescent bipolar offspring. *J Am Acad Child Adolesc Psychiatry* **39**:453–60.

Dyson WL, Barcai A (1970) Treatment of children of lithium-responding parents. *Cur Ther Res Clin Exp* **12**:286–90.

Findling RL, Youngstrom EA, Danielson CK et al (2002) Clinical decision-making using the General Behavior Inventory in Juvenile Bipolarity. *Bipolar Disord* **4**:34–42

Gaensbauer TJ, Harmon RJ, Cytryn L, McKnew DH (1984) Social and affective development in infants with a manic-depressive parent. *Am J Psychiatry* **141**:223–9.

Grigoroiu-Serbănescu M, Christodorescu D, Jipescu I, Totoescu A, Marinescu E, Ardelean V (1989) Psychopathology in children aged 10–17 of bipolar parents: psychopathology rate and correlates of the severity of the psychopathology. *J Affect Disord* **16**:167–79.

Hammen C, Burge D, Burney E, Adrian C (1990) Longitudinal study of diagnoses in children of women with unipolar and bipolar affective disorder. *Arch Gen Psychiatry* **47**:1112–17.

Klein DN, Depue RA, Slater JF (1985) Cyclothymia in the adolescent offspring of parents with bipolar affective disorder. *J Abnorm Psychol* **94**:115–27.

Lapalme M, Hodgin S, LaRoche C (1997) Children of parents with bipolar disorder: a metaanalysis of risk for mental disorders. *Can J Psychiatry* **42**:623–31.

Lewinsohn PM, Klein DN, Seeley JR (1995) Bipolar disorders in a community sample of older adolescents: prevalence, phenomenology, comorbidity, and course. *J Am Acad Child Adolesc Psychiatry* **34**:454–63.

Lish JD, Dime-Meenan S, Whybrow PC, Price RA, Hirschfeld RMA (1994) The National Depressive and Manic-Depressive Association (DMDA) survey of bipolar members. *J Affect Disord* **31**:281–94.

Manzano J, Salvador A (1993) Antecedents of severe affective (mood) disorders. Patients examined as children and adolescents and as adults. *Acta Paedopsychiatr* 56:11–18.

McKnew DH, Cytryn L, Buchsbaum MS et al (1981) Lithium in children of lithium-responding parents. *Psychiatry Res* 4:171–80.

Post RM, Weiss SRB, Leverich GS, George MS, Frye M, Ketter TA (1996) Developmental psychobiology of cyclic affective illness: implications for early therapeutic intervention. *Dev Psychopathol* 8:273–305.

Youngstrom EA, Danielson CK, Findling RL, Calabrese JR (2001) Discriminant validity of parent report of hypomanic and depressive symptoms. *Psychol Assess* 13:267–76.

Zahn-Waxler C, Mayfield A, Radke-Yarrow M, McKnew DH, Cytryn L, Davenport YB (1988) A follow-up investigation of offspring of parents with bipolar disorder. *Am J Psychiatry* **145**:506–9.

# chapter 4

# Diagnosing bipolar disorder

Bipolar disorder can be difficult to diagnose accurately in children and adolescents. However, the ability to correctly diagnose bipolar disorder in these patients is extremely important. There are many reasons that this is so. For example, as noted in Chapter 3, it has been asserted that the longer a patient with a bipolar disorder remains symptomatic and untreated, the less likely that patient is to respond to pharmacotherapy. Therefore, rapid and accurate assessment of patients with a bipolar disorder is vital so that practitioners may implement potentially life-saving treatment.

Besides missing the diagnosis of a bipolar disorder in a patient with an illness, it may be just as important to appropriately eschew giving the diagnosis of a bipolar spectrum condition to a patient who does not suffer from such a condition. Besides concerns about the stigma that is related to the illness, the diagnosis of bipolar disorder carries with it other important implications. Bipolar disorders are chronic, life-long conditions; therefore, giving a child the diagnosis of bipolar disorder means that this young person will likely require long-term treatment for a mood disorder that will almost certainly adversely affect him/her throughout the course of his/her life. Moreover, based on what is known about these illnesses, giving a patient the diagnosis of bipolar disorder generally means that the patient in question is likely to benefit optimally from chronic pharmacotherapy. This is by no means a modest implication. As discussed in later chapters of this book, many of the medications that are commonly used to treat pediatric bipolar disorders carry not only the promise of salutary effects, but they are also often associated with a significant burden. Many of the agents may lead to serious drug-related adverse events. Other compounds require the unpleasantness of phlebotomy during their administration due to the need to monitor drug levels. A substantial number of these medications are also known teratogens. This is an important consideration when making the diagnosis of bipolar disorder in adolescents and young women who may become pregnant.

As can be seen, appropriately assigning or omitting the diagnosis of a bipolar disorder carries with it substantial implications for a young person coming for psychiatric assessment. However, making a correct diagnosis of a bipolar disorder may be a challenging task.

## Difficulties with diagnosing bipolar disorder

There are several reasons why bipolar spectrum disorders may be difficult to diagnose accurately in children and adolescents. The first has to do with an appreciation of the possibility that bipolar disorders may indeed occur in young people. Until recently it has generally been accepted that bipolar disorders are rare conditions during childhood. However, recent reports suggest that young patients with bipolar disorders are commonly seen in both inpatient and outpatient settings.

Several different distinct mood states characterize bipolar disorders. Each of these mood states is associated with a particular set of symptoms and different clinical manifestations. Therefore, the clinical picture of a patient with a bipolar disorder may change substantially over a period of time. In some patients with ultradian cycling the manifestations of their illness can vary several times throughout the course of a single day.

Perhaps what has most complicated the issue of accurately diagnosing bipolar disorders in children and teenagers is a growing body of evidence that has asserted that bipolar disorders might present in a distinct fashion during the pre-adult years. The available data suggest that compared to adults higher rates of rapid cycling and irritability occur in youngsters with bipolar disorders.

With all these vicissitudes, what approaches can a clinician take to assess the possibility of a bipolar spectrum disorder in a child or teenager? What follows is a description of a systematic approach that may be employed to facilitate the accurate diagnosis of a bipolar spectrum disorder in a pediatric patient.

## The chief complaint

As any clinician who routinely works with young people knows, it is extremely uncommon for a child or teenager to request either evaluation or treatment by a mental health professional. Generally, it is the parent or guardian who seeks assistance for the child in question. However, what generally makes the accurate diagnosis of any child difficult is that there are generally only two chief complaints brought to clinicians by a youngster's parent: (i) 'My child is doing something I wish they would not do', or (ii) 'I wish my child were doing something that they are not doing'. These complaints typically focus on behaviors and externally observable features and do not focus on the internal affects and the internal perceptions of the child.

It appears that there are four common features that parents will point out to clinicians when their child does in fact have a bipolar disorder. Parents will typically describe a youngster having difficulties with one or all of the following symptoms: hyperactivity, aggression, irritability, and 'mood swings'. As can be seen, the first two of these difficulties are behavioral. Of course, bipolar disorders are not behavioral disorders per se, but children with bipolar disorders can have marked difficulties with disruptive behaviors. Table 4.1 lists the most frequent manifestations of a pediatric bipolar disorder.

## Assessing mood states

The affective states of patients with a bipolar disorder may be manic (either euphoric or irritable), depressed, mixed, or euthymic. In general,

Table 4.1  Common manifestations of pediatric bipolarity

| Aggression | Impulsivitis | Hallucinations |
|---|---|---|
| Hyperactivity | Poor frustration tolerance | Prolonged temper |
| Irritability | Grandiosity | Suicidality |
| 'Mood swings' | Sexual preoccupation | Homicidality |

young patients with bipolar disorder present with features of both depression and mania/hypomania. However, they generally do not meet full diagnostic symptom criteria for a mixed episode.

The manifest affect that appears to be most commonly appreciated in young people with bipolar disorder is irritability. When faced with a youth who has significant and pronounced irritability, a diagnosis of bipolar disorder should be considered. However, besides bipolar disorders, irritability can often be seen in depressed youngsters, youths with disruptive behavior disorders, or as a result of stressors. When a history of significantly dysfunctional mood is elicited, there are some key strategies that can be employed to assist the clinician with ruling in or ruling out a diagnosis of bipolar disorder.

The first step is to carefully attempt to identify the various mood states that are present in the youngster in question. The clinician should explore whether or not the youth that is being evaluated experiences distinct periods of irritability, elation, or depression. For those patients with mania and depression the clinician should inquire whether or not mixed episodes are also present. Are there periods when the patient's mood is apparently euthymic?

If a patient is identified who experiences mood states that might be part of a mood disorder, the next important distinction for the clinician to make with the parent and patient is to help identify whether the difficulties that are occurring are 'mood swings' and/or true 'mood episodes'. There is a group of chronically explosive, impulsive youngsters who have 'short fuses'. These youths do not experience spontaneous mood episodes that are characteristic of affective conditions.

Moreover, these youths do not develop the other symptoms of a mood episode during these explosive outbursts. For example, when irritated or angered, although they may lash out aggressively, these youths will not develop the decreased need for sleep, grandiosity, or increased loquaciousness that characterize a manic episode. Many of these youths generally meet diagnostic symptom criteria for a primary diagnosis of a disruptive behavior disorder. Conversely, it should be remembered that while youths are experiencing an affective episode, they might appear to be quite explosive and unpredictable. The key distinction is what came first, the mood or the event that precipitated the behavior. Often this is the most difficult part of the evaluation. Table 4.2 lists the keys to reaching an accurate diagnosis of pediatric bipolar disorder.

If spontaneous mood episodes are identified, it can be most helpful to review and consider the natural history of these affective states. We have generally found it quite useful for parents and/or youngsters to complete life charting with respect to the child's mood states as part of the assessment process. By definition, bipolar disorder is a cyclic condition. Although parents and children may initially report an unwavering course of illness without cycling, after being taught the life charting method (LCM) most parents of children and adolescents with bipolar disorder will indeed report a cyclic condition.

## Assessing family history

There is a great deal of evidence to support the idea that genetics plays a role in the development of bipolar disorder. For this reason, a careful, thorough family history may be useful when assessing a youth in whom a bipolar disorder is being considered. Unfortunately, there is evidence that bipolar disorder is not always promptly or accurately diagnosed in adults. Thus, simply asking whether or not a family member has been diagnosed with bipolar disorder or 'manic depression' is often not adequate.

Careful attention to mood episodes in parents, siblings, grandparents, aunts, and uncles can frequently be quite enlightening. It is not

Table 4.2  Keys to diagnosing accurately pediatric bipolar disorders

1. **Assess/identify mood states**
   Depressed
      Sad
      Irritable
   Manic/hypomanic
      Elated/elevated
      Irritable
   Mixed
   Euthymic

2. **Characterize mood states**
   Spontaneous or only precipitated?

3. **Take a detailed family history**

4. **Assess longitudinal course**
   Life Charting Method (LCM) may be helpful

5. **Assess time course of other symptoms**
   Disruptive behaviors
   Psychosis
   Anxiety
   Substance abuse

6. **Rule out general medical conditions**

7. **Rule out medication-induced mood states**

8. **Carefully assess environmental factors**

uncommon for a thorough clinician, during the course of an assessment of a young person with bipolar disorder, to identify a patient's family member as possibly also suffering from this condition.

## Assessing disruptive behaviors

When faced with a child or teenager with substantial difficulties with hyperactivity or aggressive behavior, the possibility of a bipolar disorder should be considered. However, it should be remembered that the symptom of hyperactivity or restlessness could occur in a large number of psychiatric disorders. These include attention-deficit hyperactivity disorder (ADHD), depression, anxiety disorders, substance abuse, and psychotic illnesses. In addition, disruptive behaviors may be the result of environmental stressors that are either chronic or acute.

When evaluating a patient with significant dysfunctional hyperactivity, it is important for the clinician to consider the possibility that the manifest restlessness that is present may be due to a bipolar disorder. To assess for this, the key issue to be considered is not whether substantial hyperactivity is present. The main focus of the evaluation should be on whether or not hyperactivity, impulsivity, inattention and aggression become exacerbated during spontaneous mood episodes in which the other symptoms that define these mood states are also present.

## Psychosis

Patients with bipolar disorders often have symptoms of psychosis. However, it appears as if most young people with bipolar disorder who describe psychotic symptoms are not truly psychotic. For example, it seems as if the majority of juvenile patients with psychotic symptoms may occasionally 'hear noises' or periodically 'see shadows at night' while not having prominent hallucinations or delusions.

However, young patients with bipolar disorder can indeed suffer from full-blown psychotic episodes. When faced with any youngster with a psychotic episode, the diagnoses of bipolar disorder or schizoaffective disorder should be considered. If it is clear that the patient in question has a disorder with a prominent psychotic component and also suffers from mood episodes, it is important to ascertain when in the course of the condition the youngster has both the psychosis and the affective disturbances.

In youngsters with mood disorders with psychotic features, the psychosis typically occurs during the periods of time when their mood disturbances are most prevalent. Conversely, if a patient is suffering from schizoaffective disorder, psychosis will be present even during those times when the affective components of the illness are quiescent. Accurately making the distinction between bipolar disorder and schizoaffective disorder is important as both conditions may differ in outcome and means of treatment.

## Anxiety

Patients with bipolar disorders may appear quite anxious at times. There is evidence that young patients with bipolar disorder may seem as if they are suffering from an anxiety disorder. Indeed, these youths may initially be diagnosed with an anxiety disorder. However, it appears as if the majority of juveniles with bipolar disorders do not meet diagnostic symptom criteria for an anxiety disorder per se.

During the manic or hypomanic phase of the illness, youths may appear tense and display repetitive behaviors. These youths may appear to suffer from generalized anxiety disorder or obsessive-compulsive disorder. In addition, during the depressive phase of the condition, children and teenagers may seem to be generally anxious, phobic, or socially avoidant.

Youths with bipolar disorders and prominent symptoms of anxiety will have their anxiety wax and wane with their mood states, while those with a primary anxiety disorder are in general chronically anxious.

## Substance abuse

It is an unfortunate reality that teenagers with bipolar disorders are at high risk for substance abuse. A teenager who is acting in an unusual fashion or is manifesting disruptive behaviors should have a toxicology screen obtained or have a substance abuse assessment initiated. However, it is important to remember that teenagers with positive toxicology screens and substance abuse disorders may suffer from a variety of neuropsychiatric illnesses. For this reason, when a teenager has an identified substance abuse problem, a thorough assessment for the presence of a mood disorder should be considered. Conversely, when a young person is diagnosed with a bipolar disorder, the possibility of a substance abuse disorder also needs to be kept in mind.

Finally it should be recalled that symptoms of mania or depression could occur during periods of intoxication or withdrawal from several substances of abuse. For this reason, a careful review of the longitudinal course of symptom expression and its relationship to the abuse of substances is needed when faced with a youngster who might be suffering from a mood disorder, a substance abuse disorder, or both.

## General medical conditions

There are many general medical conditions that can mimic symptoms of mania, depression, or psychosis. These include metabolic disorders (especially those involving the thyroid, parathyroid and adrenal glands), neurological conditions, infectious diseases, and medications (including stimulants and antidepressants). The possibility of a general medical condition or a medication-related disorder should always be considered when faced with a youngster with symptoms of bipolar disorder.

## Summary

Patients with bipolar disorder generally present with both significant behavioral difficulties and problematic mood states. When faced with youngsters with these concerns, it is important for the clinician to consider the possibility that the child in question may suffer from a bipolar spectrum disorder. To accurately make the diagnosis of a bipolar illness to a youngster it is essential for the clinician to be familiar with the differential diagnosis of bipolar disorders. These include a wide variety of other psychiatric illnesses, non-syndromal mood or behavioral states, and general medical conditions but it is important for bipolar illness to be a diagnosis of exclusion or last resort.

Besides carefully considering the extensive differential diagnosis of bipolar disorder when faced with a youngster with mood and/or behavioral difficulties, two key approaches appear to be most useful. The first includes a careful appreciation of the longitudinal course of the condition. Patients do not develop bipolar disorders overnight. These conditions gradually unfold, 'mature', and become more problematic over time. Moreover, as bipolar disorders, by definition, are episodic conditions, the ability to identify accurately spontaneous changes between mood states is vital before considering the diagnosis of bipolar disorder in a young person. Tracking the longitudinal course of the illness with both retrospective and prospective life charting may be quite helpful in this regard.

There are other aspects to the medical history that should also be carefully considered when faced with a child or teenager who might be suffering from a bipolar disorder. Genetics is a well-established risk factor for bipolar disorders. Considering the fact that bipolar disorder may not be accurately or promptly diagnosed in adults, simply asking whether anyone in the family has been diagnosed with bipolar disorder is not enough. A meticulous family history can be very informative. Finally, as there are many symptom clusters that may become manifest during the course of a bipolar illness, accurately identifying affective states and their relationships to these other symptom groups may be quite important.

In short, making an accurate diagnosis of bipolar disorder in a child or teenager is often a difficult task. Factors that contribute to this problem include the numerous ways in which these conditions may present and the fact that the most overt manifestations may be those of other neuropsychiatric conditions. However a careful consideration of the longitudinal course of illness coupled with a thorough family history can facilitate the accurate assessment of a young patient who may be suffering from a bipolar disorder.

It should also be noted that another factor that complicates the accurate assessment and diagnosis of pediatric bipolarity is the high rates of psychiatric co-morbidity that are seen in young patients with these conditions. What these co-morbidities are and how to assess them carefully are considered in more detail in Chapter 5.

## Further reading

Carlson GA (1990) Annontation: child and adolescent mania – diagnostic considerations. *J Child Psychol Psychiatr* **31**:331–41.

Findling RL, Calabrese JR (2000) Rapid-cycling bipolar disorder in children. *Am J Psychiatry* **15**:1526–7.

Findling RL, Schulz SC, Kashani JH, Harlan E (2001) *Psychotic Disorders in Children and Adolescents*. Thousand Oaks: Sage Publications.

Geller B, Luby J (1997) Child and adolescent bipolar disorder: a review of the past 10 years. *J Am Acad Child Adolesc Psychiatry* **36**:1168–76.

Geller B, Zimmerman B, Williams M et al (2000a) Diagnostic characteristics of 93 cases of prepubertal and early adolescent bipolar disorder phenotype by gender, puberty and comorbid attention deficit hyperactivity disorder. *J Child Adolesc Psychopharmacol* **10**:157–64.

Geller B, Zimmerman B, Williams M et al (2000b) Six-month stability and outcome of a prepubertal and early adolescent bipolar disorder phenotype. *J Child Adolesc Psychopharmacol* **10**:165–73.

Hutto B (1999) The symptoms of depression in endocrine disorders. *CNS Spectrums* **4**:51–61.

Larson EW, Richelson E (1988) Organic causes of mania. *Mayo Clin Proc* **63**:906–12.

Leverich GS, Post RM (1988) Life charting of affective disorders. *CNS Spectrums* **3**:21–37.

Pies RW (1994) Medical 'mimics' of depression. *Psychiatr Ann* **24**:519–20.

# chapter 5

# Psychiatric co-morbidity

As discussed in previous chapters, accurately making a diagnosis of a bipolar spectrum disorder in a child or adolescent can be quite a difficult task. This is because bipolar disorders may present in a variety of diverse ways in these young patients. What further complicates either correctly assigning or eschewing a diagnosis of a bipolar spectrum disorder in a young person is the consistent observation that high rates of psychiatric co-morbidity seem to occur in children and adolescents with bipolar disorders. Although definitive epidemiological data do not exist, it appears that significant psychiatric co-morbidity occurs in at least three-quarters of young patients with bipolar disorders.

Since more than one psychiatric syndrome is often present in these children and teenagers, once a clinician is confident that a young person does suffer from a bipolar disorder, it is essential to examine diligently whether or not other psychiatric conditions are present. This is because the accurate identification of co-morbid neuropsychiatric disorders may be quite important when developing a treatment plan for these young patients.

The most common psychiatric co-morbidities seen in pediatric patients with bipolar disorders appear to be: attention-deficit/hyperactivity disorder (ADHD), oppositional defiant disorder (OpDD), and conduct disorder (CD). It appears that more than half of patients with juvenile bipolar disorder also suffer from at least one of these three conditions. Other co-morbidities that frequently occur in these patients include

Table 5.1  Common co-morbidities in pediatric bipolar disorder

Disruptive disorders
   Attention-deficit/hyperactivity disorder
   Oppositional defiant disorder
   Conduct disorder
Anxiety disorders
Substance abuse disorders

anxiety and substance abuse disorders. Table 5.1 lists the most commonly seen psychiatric co-morbidities in young people with a bipolar spectrum disorder.

## Assessing for co-morbidities

Many of the psychiatric disorders that occur as co-morbidities in young patients with a bipolar spectrum disorder can mistakenly be perceived as manifestations of the bipolar illness itself. This is because the presentation of these other conditions can have a similar appearance to the symptoms of the affective illness. For example, youngsters with either ADHD or hypomania may appear hyperkinetic. Similarly, youths who are in the depressed phase of their illness may appear quite anxious. How then can a clinician attempt to identify accurately psychiatric co-morbidities in young patients with bipolar disorders?

As noted in Chapter 4, during the assessment of a child or adolescent for whom a bipolar spectrum disorder is suspected, it is important for the clinician to identify whether or not spontaneous manic, depressed, or mixed states are present. These mood states are generally more readily identified when they are compared to the youth's relatively 'good periods' in which parents and youngsters will note that the child's mood is 'in the middle'. It is our experience that more often than not these periods of euthymia (albeit frequently brief) can often be accurately

Table 5.2 Steps to co-morbidity assessment

Always consider the possibility of co-morbidity
   One or more co-morbid diagnoses are possible
Take a careful longitudinal history
   Life charting method (LCM) may be useful
Identify behavior and functioning during affective episodes
Identify behavior and functioning during euthymia
Examine whether other conditions are present during euthymia

identified. Using the life charting method (LCM) can often facilitate this task.

After this is accomplished, the child's emotional state and psycho-social functioning during the identified period of neutral mood can then be meticulously considered and accurately described. Once a clear clinical picture of the youth during euthymic periods can be ascertained, then the presence or absence of psychiatric co-morbidities can most appropriately be made. Table 5.2 lists the steps that are most useful in psychiatric co-morbidity assessment.

The early identification of psychiatric co-morbidities has important practical clinical implications. For example, a youth may appear to be oppositional during periods of depression due to profound irritability. However, during periods of euthymia, it may be learned during the assessment process that the patient may still have significant difficulties with defiance. If a parent's key motivation for bringing the child for a clinical assessment relates to the youth's oppositionality, a parent might not consider a 'successful' treatment with a thymoleptic agent meaningful if the youngster's mood improves and the patient remains defiant.

In short, optimal treatment of a child with a bipolar spectrum disorder must address both the affective illness as well as the psychiatric co-morbidities. For this reason, the clinician must carefully evaluate the possibility of psychiatric co-morbidities in these patients.

Ideally, the presence or absence of concomitant psychiatric disorders can be made during the assessment process. This is not always feasible. It may be difficult for some parents and youths to identify and describe a patient's psychosocial functioning during euthymic periods. In such cases it may be useful for the clinician to review with the patient and the patient's family the high likelihood that psychiatric co-morbidities are present in young people with bipolar disorders. This way, as the treatment of the affective disorder gets under way and the patient's mood stabilizes, both the patient and the clinician can be watchful for the presence or absence of psychiatric co-morbidities that will also need to be addressed to provide optimal patient care.

## Disruptive behavior disorders: a heuristic example

The available evidence suggests that the most common psychiatric co-morbidities for patients with bipolar illnesses are ADHD and the disruptive behavior disorders. The diagnosis of co-morbid ADHD is commonly assigned to young patients with bipolar illnesses. In fact, it appears as if an earlier age at onset of a bipolar spectrum disorder is associated with a higher risk for co-morbid ADHD. Although youths with a bipolar disorder may suffer from either the hyperactive/impulsive or inattentive type of ADHD, it seems as if the most common form of ADHD seen in young people with a bipolar illness is the combined type.

Considering its high prevalence, it is not surprising that the psychiatric co-morbidity of ADHD in youths with bipolar illness has received the greatest amount of attention from both clinicians as well as investigators. Another reason why the co-morbidity of ADHD and bipolar disorder has received so much attention is because it often can be quite difficult distinguishing between these two conditions. Both of these syndromes are characterized by symptoms of restlessness, impulsiveness, and distractibility.

Similarly, there is also a significant amount of symptom overlap between OpDD and bipolar illnesses. Youngsters with both disorders can appear irritable and surly. Moreover, young patients who are grandiose may appear defiant to adults, as these youths feel as if they know what is right, and feel that they do not need to listen to anyone. In a similar fashion, young patients with bipolar illness can become quite aggressive and engage in antisocial acts. For this reason, many youths with bipolar disorders may appear to be suffering from co-morbid CD.

For these reasons when evaluating a disruptive youngster it is important to consider the possibility of a bipolar disorder. However, it appears that the majority of patients with a disruptive behavior disorder do not suffer from a co-morbid bipolar disorder. Whether to assign or eschew a diagnosis of a bipolar disorder in these patients should be based on a meticulous longitudinal history in which the presence of mood states is carefully considered (see Chapter 4).

The following is an illustrative case vignette:

The patient was a 12-year-old female who was brought in by her mother for evaluation of 'depression'. The patient was initially diagnosed with ADHD at the age of 3 by a pediatric neurologist due to difficulties with restlessness, aggression, and difficulty following through on instructions at both pre-school and at home. After numerous unsuccessful attempts at behavior modification over the next 5 years, the patient's pediatrician began a therapeutic trial of methylphenidate due to persistent difficulties. Although the patient's deportment improved substantially with pharmacotherapy, the patient's mother felt the patient 'wasn't herself' while taking the psychostimulant. For this reason, pharmacotherapy was discontinued after about 6 months.

Approximately 2 years prior to this current evaluation, the patient spontaneously became 'moody'. She would either isolate herself from other children or would be 'bossy' with them. This significantly affected her peer relationships. In addition, although the patient had consistent difficulties with behavior at school, she had generally achieved academically at the Merit Roll level. After her 'moodiness' developed, her grades began to decline markedly. At home she became more defiant with her mother and began to bully her young sibling. Other clinicians made diagnoses of both OpDD and CD. A behavioral modification program was initiated, but it failed to ameliorate the patient's difficulties.

During the present evaluation, the patient's mother described a gradual development and worsening of the patient's 'depression' characterized by spontaneous periods of irritability over the past 2 years. It was also ascertained that the patient would have periods of time (usually lasting several days) during which she would become profoundly sad and would isolate herself in her room. During these periods, the patient would proclaim that 'no one liked her', and that she wished she had never been born. Like the other mood states, these periods also occurred spontaneously. During other times the patient was more aggressive, profoundly overactive, and extremely talkative. The patient's mother remarked that her daughter appeared to 'not need sleep' during these times. In addition, periods of pronounced mood elevation were identified during which 'everything seemed funny' and the patient would talk so quickly that she was difficult to understand. During these episodes that would last several days, the patient would speak of plans to become a famous actress. The patient did not appear to be using drugs or alcohol. Interestingly enough the patient's mother also noted that there were brief periods of time when the patient was 'her old self'. During these periods, the patient was able to get along well with others again and would not bully her sibling.

The patient had a family history significant for 'depression' in her mother. The father's whereabouts and history were not known. Based on the results of the assessment, a diagnosis of a bipolar disorder was made for the patient.

As can be seen from this brief vignette, young patients with a bipolar spectrum disorder may also suffer from co-morbid ADHD or disruptive behavior disorders. In this youngster's case, a diagnosis of ADHD seems appropriate. This is because the patient consistently had a history of persistent, pervasive, and problematic difficulties with restlessness, impulsiveness, and distractibility that occurred during periods of neutral mood. However, based on this history, a diagnosis of OpDD and CD would not be appropriate because it appears as if the difficulties associated with oppositionality and aggression and bullying only occurred during mood episodes.

This vignette highlights the need for meticulous longitudinal assessment regarding symptom development for a patient in whom a diagnosis of bipolar disorder might be suspected. A similar approach may also be considered when faced with a youth with other symptoms (such as anxiety, psychotic, or substance abuse difficulties).

## Summary

Definitive rates for these co-morbidities have still not been established. However, it appears that high rates of psychiatric co-morbidity are present in juvenile bipolarity. At present it seems as if the majority of youths with bipolar disorder also suffer from ADHD or a co-morbid disruptive behavior disorder. Because there seems to be such high rates of co-morbidity, the possibility that other psychiatric diagnoses might be present should always be considered when the diagnosis of bipolar disorder has been assigned to a young person. Accurate identification of co-morbid conditions can allow for the development of a treatment plan that more comprehensively addresses the needs of the patient.

## Further reading

Biederman J, Faraone S, Mick E et al (1996) Attention-deficit hyperactivity disorder and juvenile mania: an overlooked comorbidity? *J Am Acad Child Adolesc Psychiatry* **35**:997–1008.

Carlson GA (1998) Mania and ADHD: comorbidity or confusion. *J Affect Disord* **51**:177–87.

Findling RL, Gracious BL, McNamara NK, Youngstrom EA, Demeter CA, Branicky LA, Calabrese JR (2001) Rapid continuous cycling and psychiatric co-morbidity in pediatric bipolar I disorder. *Bipolar Disorders* **3**:202–10.

Kutcher S, Robertson HA, Bird D (1998) Premorbid functioning in adolescent onset bipolar I disorder: a preliminary report from an ongoing study. *J Affect Disord* **51**:137–44.

McElroy SL, Strakowski SM, West SA, Keck PE, Jr., McConville BJ (1997) Phenomenology of adolescent and adult mania in hospitalized patients with bipolar disorder. *Am J Psychiatry* **154**:44–9.

Milberger S, Biederman J, Faraone SV, Murphy J, Tsuang MT (1995) Attention deficit hyperactivity disorder and comorbid disorders: issues of overlapping symptoms. *Am J Psychiatry* **152**:1793–9.

West SA, Strakowski SM, Sax KW, McElroy SL, Keck PE, Jr., McConville BJ (1996) Phenomenology and comorbidity of adolescents hospitalized for the treatment of acute mania. *Biol Psychiatry* **39**:458–60.

Wozniak J, Biederman J, Richards JA (2001) Diagnostic and therapeutic dilemmas in the management of pediatric-onset bipolar disorder. *J Clin Psychiatry* **62**(suppl 14):10–15.

# chapter 6

# Causes and mechanisms of bipolar illness: a focus on childhood onset

Although the precise causes and mechanisms involved in the onset and progression of bipolar illness have not been conclusively identified, much evidence is accumulating about the general types of processes involved. We know that bipolar illness runs strongly in families, with genetics playing a role in the vulnerability to illness onset in approximately 50% of adult patients with bipolar illness. It is likely that genetic vulnerability plays an even greater role in childhood-onset bipolar disorder, although a substantial number of patients with bipolar illness do not have a family history of bipolar illness in their first-degree relatives, so other non-hereditary mechanisms must also be considered.

Different biological mechanisms may also be involved in different stages of illness evolution. Thus, the occurrence of early stressors may increase sensitivity to subsequent stressors and the associated development of high levels of cortisol during depressive episodes. In those who are highly genetically predisposed or following many affective episodes, bouts of illness may begin to occur in the absence of psychosocial stressors. In depression, biochemical and structural abnormalities have been found that are associated with decreased neural activity in the frontal cortex, as well as alterations in the function of the limbic areas of the brain which are thought to be most intimately involved in the regulation of emotion. Depressive episodes may thus be the result of deficient excitation or increased inhibition, whereas the opposite might occur in mania. To the extent that the illness tends to be recurrent, and neurobiological alterations associated with each episode further increase the vulnerability to new recurrences, the importance of the early institution of long-term prophylactic treatment becomes increasingly clear. It is this preliminary conceptual formulation of illness progression that is outlined in this chapter.

## The genetics of bipolar illness

The genetic vulnerability associated with bipolar illness is most evident from studies of identical twins compared with fraternal twins. Identical twins share the same genes and thus should have the same illnesses, to the extent that there are genetically mediated factors. Identical twins are highly concordant for bipolar illness (both having the illness between 40 and 70% of the time, i.e. a rate much higher than other psychiatric illnesses), whereas the concordance is less than half that for fraternal twins (who do not share the same genes, but do share the same environment) (Craddock and Jones 1999).

These data for identical twins are supported by familial studies indicating that when there is a positive family history of bipolar illness in first-degree relatives, risk in their children increases considerably from about 1% of the normal population to about 10–20% (Craddock and Jones 1999). Thus, one in five children are likely to develop bipolar illness based on this type of vulnerability. However, when there is bipolar illness on one side of the family and either unipolar or bipolar illness on the other side, the risk of a child developing some type of affective illness (either unipolar or bipolar) then increases to about 70%. This is because the risks appear to be additive or multiplicative because of what is thought to be a very complex and polygenic (multi-caused) basis of the hereditary vulnerability, as well as that from the environment. Thus, several vulnerability genes may come from one side of the family and converge with other vulnerability genes from the other side of the family.

Not only is the risk evident from family studies, but it is also apparent in the opposite direction. That is, if one studies first-degree relatives of children with early-onset bipolar disorder, more relatives are affected than in those with adolescent-onset and, especially, adult-onset disorder. These data suggest that a greater background of genetic vulnerability is associated with the increased risk of childhood-onset bipolar illness.

## The generational or cohort effects

Recently there has been a description of what is technically called the 'cohort' effect, meaning that each generation born since World War I appears to have an increased rate as well as an earlier age of onset of unipolar and bipolar illness than the previous generation (Gershon et al 1987). There has been much speculation about the potential mechanisms involved in the increased rate and earlier onset of affective disorders in the general population.

Whatever reasons emerge to account for this dramatic trend, it has been a factor in a very considerable change in recognizing affective illness in children. Some 20–30 years ago it was argued that childhood-onset depression may not exist, and mania in children was virtually unheard of. Today, both depressive and manic mood states are common, and recurrent depressions and bipolar illness can begin in the very first years of life in highly predisposed individuals (Figure 6.1).

Some people have wondered whether the increased recognition of rapid mood fluctuations in children is partially attributable to the increasing use of psychomotor stimulants for the treatment of attention-deficit hyperactivity disorder (ADHD). This is of some concern since many investigators have noted that there is a high co-morbidity of ADHD with bipolar illness (Biederman et al 1996), and that the ADHD cannot be treated adequately until the bipolar illness is first treated with a mood stabilizer. In the potentially bipolar child, if one uses stimulants alone, this might exacerbate mood fluctuations.

### Genetic anticipation

Genetic anticipation refers to the findings in some genetic illnesses that a decrease in the age of onset may occur in successive generations. This

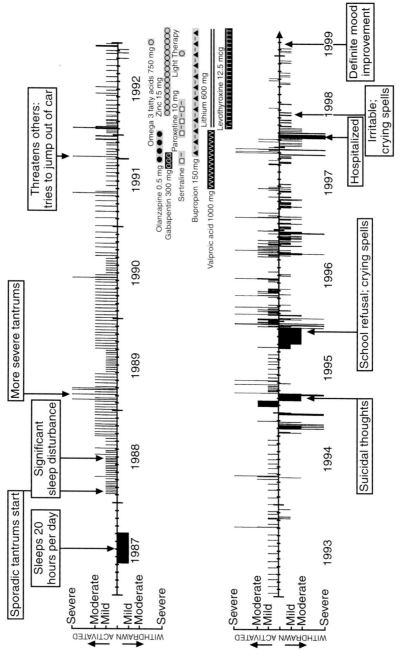

**Figure 6.1** 'Kiddie' life chart of a 12-year-old child with affective dysfunction from the first year of life.

has been found to be true for neurological illnesses such as Huntington's disease, spinal cerebellar degeneration, fragile X syndrome, and other neurodegenerative disorders (Li and el Mallakh 1997). In the case of Huntington's disease, it was found that the defect that causes this illness (associated with progressive dementia and involuntary motor movements) is in a single protein called huntingtin. The genetic code for this protein has multiple triple-repeat sequences in a row that code for the amino acid glutamine. If an individual has fewer than 40 of these triple-repeat sequences, Huntington's disease does not occur. If there are about 47 or more, the individual will develop Huntington's disease late in life. With a very large number of triple-repeats, e.g. 60 or 70, the illness may be associated with a very early onset (even in childhood).

When the sperm and egg cells of individuals with the Huntington's disease gene reproduce themselves, there is some tendency for the number of triple-repeat sequences to expand. Thus, people who might be destined to develop Huntington's disease relatively late in life because they were born with approximately 50 triple-repeat sequences, may have children with 60–70 triple-repeats in a row, rendering the huntingtin protein highly dysfunctional and associated with a very early onset of the illness in these people's children.

This expansion of the triple-repeat sequence is what is referred to as genetic anticipation and indicates that there are mechanisms within the replication of an individual's reproductive cells (egg or sperm) that can increase the degree of defect in some single-gene illnesses from one generation to the next. Although not consistently demonstrated, several investigative groups have suggested that there are triple-repeat sequences associated with bipolar illness, and there may be evidence of a genetic anticipation mechanism whereby the next generation may have an illness onset as great as 10 years earlier than their parents (Mendlewicz et al 1997). However, it is also possible that an earlier onset of illness is only manifestation of the general cohort effect and could be associated with a variety of other factors that are not necessarily related to genetic inheritance (Lange and McInnes 2002).

## Searching for genetic vulnerability factors

Over the past decade there has been an increasing effort to identify the genetic changes that may increase vulnerability to bipolar illness. One of the most promising leads has been found on the short arm of chromosome 18 with the initial findings of Berrettini et al (1994), which were replicated and extended by DePaulo and colleagues (Stine et al 1995; McMahon et al 1997). These investigators noted that inheritance with a marker on chromosome 18 was associated with bipolar II illness on the father's side of the family and that maternal transmission of the illness was not associated with such a vulnerability factor on this chromosome. These findings suggest that one should search further in this region of chromosome 18 to identify precisely the nature of the molecular alteration involved. However, even when the general area of the short arm of chromosome 4 was discovered to convey vulnerability to Huntington's disease (which shows a much simpler pattern of genetic inheritance involving a single gene), it still required approximately a decade before the actual protein defect was isolated and found to be the huntingtin protein.

Thus, in the case of bipolar illness, it is likely to take as long or longer for this possible gene defect on chromosome 18 to be discovered, and it is highly likely to be one of a great many vulnerability factors, much like that now evident in diabetes and in cancer. For example, in the development of colon cancer, there are initial stages of increased proliferation and cell multiplication before a full-blown tumor is developed, and, with further evolution of the tumor, a cancerous tumor may develop in a single location characterized by more aggressive cell types that are clearly abnormal upon microscopic examination. In later stages, the tumor cells may metastasize and break away from the primary site and, with this transition, become resistant to treatment. This progression, in terms of colon cancer, involves a series of mutations that not only increase cellular proliferation, but also disable normal tumor suppressor factors. If an individual is born into a family that already has a genetic vulnerability, for example, based on loss of a tumor suppressor factor, they may be at particularly high risk for earlier onset of the disorder because fewer mutations are necessary to produce the full-blown illness.

We believe that the same types of illness progression occur in bipolar illness, with a certain number of alterations in gene expression occurring based on heredity and another group based on life experiences, stresses, and the experience of multiple episodes of affective dysregulation (Figure 6.2). However, instead of these environmental events causing irreversible mutations as in cancer, in bipolar illness they would only tend to cause transient biochemical alterations; that is, a change only in what genes are expressed and to what degree. Therefore, when the vulnerability factors for bipolar illness are ultimately identified, they are not likely to provide the same definitive information that comes with knowing whether or not one has inherited the single gene defect of Huntington's disease. In this case, one knows with a fair degree of certainty whether or not they will eventually get the illness.

In contrast, in the case of multiply determined or polygenic illnesses such as heart disease or bipolar illness, the inheritance of a given susceptibility gene would have only a small effect and would not necessarily mean that an individual will become ill. However, the identification of a series of small-effect susceptibility genes for bipolar illness may not only help to understand the mechanisms of illness generation and progression, but could also eventually help identify the treatments to which a patient may best respond.

# The importance of stressors and episodes in bipolar illness

## Stress sensitization

Kraepelin (1921) first proposed the concept that the first episodes of mania or depression are often precipitated by psychosocial stressors, but that with sufficient numbers of recurrences lesser degrees of stress are required, and episodes begin to emerge more spontaneously or autonomously. In a meta analysis we found that there was a substantial literature validating this concept (Post 1992). New data are highly supportive of this stress sensitization perspective. Data in the Stanley Foun-

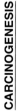
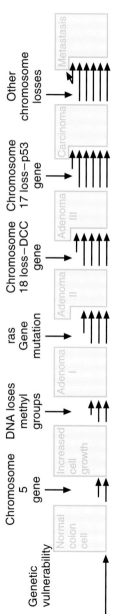
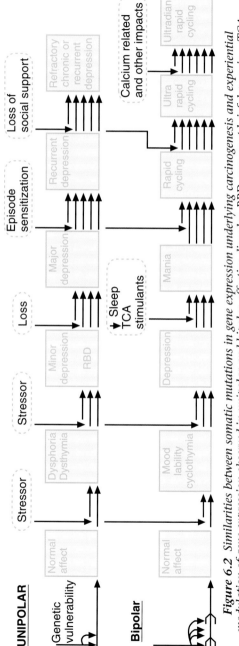

*Figure 6.2 Similarities between somatic mutations in gene expression underlying carcinogenesis and experiential modulation of gene expression observed in unipolar and bipolar affective disorder. RBD, recurrent brief depression; TCA, tricyclic antidepressant.*

dation Bipolar Network (SFBN) are also consistent with an important role of early stressful life events in conveying a long-lasting vulnerability to stressors and their ability to trigger episodes. In a study of more than 600 patients in the SFBN, those with a history of early extreme environmental adversity (i.e. physical or sexual abuse in childhood or adolescence) had an earlier onset of bipolar illness, a more pernicious course, and more Axis I, Axis II, and Axis III co-morbidities (Leverich et al 2001).

## Episode sensitization

These observations are taken in the context of the general tendency for the frequency of episodes to accelerate over time. Again, Kraepelin was among the first to document that the 'well-interval' between the first and second episodes tended to be longer than the interval between the second and third and other successive episodes (Figure 6.3). This has also now been well validated in the literature. However, this does not imply that the tendency for progression cannot be stopped with successful treatment. It is, rather, only that the general course of the illness, with its extreme varieties of cyclic presentation, is one that tends to go in the direction of cycle acceleration if not otherwise treated.

Kessing and associates in Denmark have provided the best documentation of this phenomenon of episode sensitization, i.e. that 'episodes

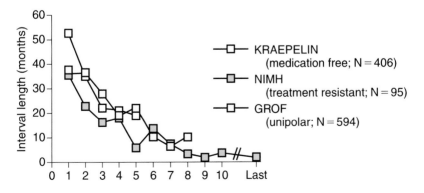

**Figure 6.3** *Decreasing well intervals between successive episodes in the emergence of recurrent affective illness in three different study samples.*

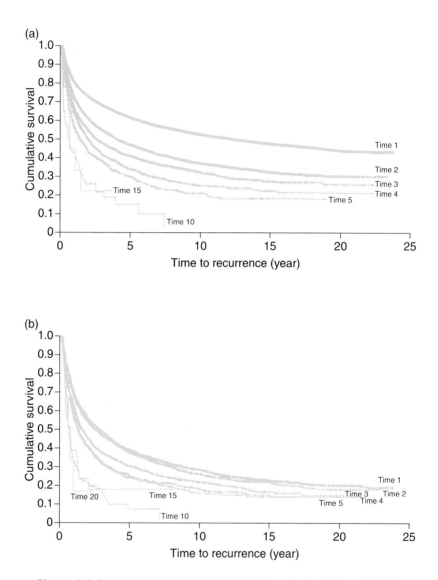

**Figure 6.4** *Recurrence at successive episodes in unipolar (top) and bipolar (bottom) affective disorder. Cumulative survival (probability of remaining well) was calculated using the Kaplan–Meier method for estimation with censored observations. For both unipolar (a) and bipolar (b) patients, time to recurrence (labeled Time 1, Time 2, etc.) decreased with the number of previous episodes. (Reprinted with permission from Kessing LV et al (1998)* Br J Psychiatry *172:23–8.)*

beget episodes' (Figure 6.4). They observed that in both unipolar and bipolar hospitalizations, the best predictor of the incidence and time course to relapse was the number of prior episodes. These data were observed in 20,350 patients carefully tracked in the Danish case registry and provide further confirmation of Kraepelin's original formulation of cycle acceleration as a function of episode recurrence (Kessing et al 1998).

These kinds of data have been synthesized in the concepts that recurrent stressors and episodes can both predispose an individual to an increased vulnerability to future episodes in a long-lasting fashion (Figure 6.5). For either stressor or episode sensitization to occur, there has to be some kind of underlying memory-like mechanism conveying these long-term changes (Figure 6.6). Given these general tendencies for the course of bipolar illness to accelerate over time and move from psychosocially triggered to spontaneous episodes, we became very interested in the phenomena of sensitization and kindling in animals as models of neuronal learning and memory that had certain parallels with the evolution of affective illness.

## The kindling model

In kindling, repeated intermittent subthreshold stimulation of a given region of the brain in rodents eventually leads to full-blown seizures, and with sufficient numbers of these triggered seizures they begin to occur spontaneously, i.e. the animal begins to have seizures even when its brain is not stimulated (Figure 6.7). The neurobiology of this neuronal learning process is beginning to be revealed at the level of long-term changes in gene expression of neurotransmitters, receptors, and nerve growth (or neurotrophic) factors, as well as in the micro-structure of the synapse and nerve cell survival and cell death. These alterations probably occur on the basis of changes in gene transcription (Figures 6.6 and 6.8). That is, whatever one's genetic inheritance, genes continue to be turned on and off not only throughout the development of the nervous system, but also in response to stressors, life events, and even

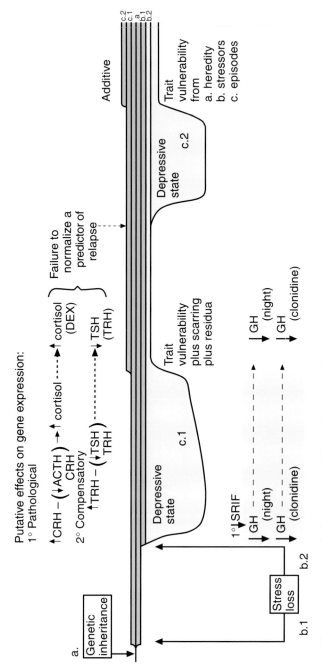

**Figure 6.5** *Accumulating experiential genetic vulnerability in recurrent affective illness. Initial stressors that might not be sufficient to trigger the full neurobiological concomitants of a depressive episode (STATE) may nonetheless leave behind biological (TRAIT) vulnerabilities (shaded center line) to further alterations. The state of depression with its associated peptide and hormonal increases (top) and decreases (bottom) may then leave behind additional trait vulnerabilities and residua. ACTH, adrenocorticotropic hormone; GH, growth hormone; DEX, dexamethasone; TRH, thyrotropin-releasing hormone; SRIF, somatostatin; TSH, thyroid-stimulating hormone.*

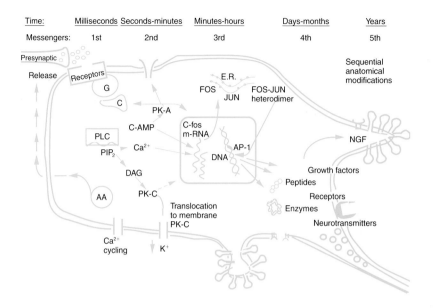

**Figure 6.6** *Neural mechanisms of synaptic plasticity, short- and long-term memory. This schematic of a cell illustrates how transient synaptic events induced by external stimuli can exert longer-lasting effects on neuronal excitability and microstructure of the brain via a cascade of effects involving alterations in gene transcription. Neurotransmitters activate receptors and second-messenger systems, which then induce immediate early genes (IEGs) such as* c-fos *and* c-jun. *Fos and Jun proteins are synthesized on the endoplasmic reticulum (E.R.) and then bind to DNA to further alter the transcription of late effector genes (LEGs) and other regulatory factors, the effects of which could last for months or years. PLC, phospholipase C; PIP$_2$, phosphatidyl inositol 4,5-biphosphate; AA, arachidonic acid; DAG, diacyglycerol; PKC, protein kinase-C; AP-1, activator protein 1 (binding site on DNA); PK-A, protein kinase-A.*

normal processes of learning and memory. The kindling formulation has also helped us to conceptualize that some of the changes in gene transcription (Figure 6.9) are related to the primary pathophysiology of kindling (i.e. the 'bad guys' of the long-term kindled memory trace), whereas others are secondary, compensatory, transient anticonvulsant adaptations (i.e. the 'good guys' trying to prevent further seizures).

It is of some interest that thyrotropin-releasing hormone (TRH) is not only a likely endogenous antidepressant in affective illness, but also an

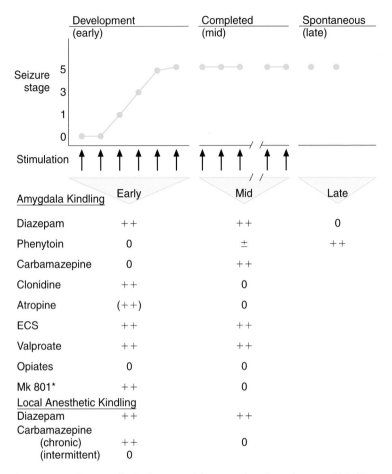

**Figure 6.7** *Pharmacological responsivity as a function of stage of kindling. Top: Schematic illustration of the evolution of kindled seizures. Initial stimulation (development) are associated with progressively increasing after-discharge duration (not shown) and behavioral seizure stage. Subsequent stimulations (completed) produce reliable generalized motor seizures. Spontaneous seizures emerge after sufficient numbers of triggered seizures have been generated (usually >100). Bottom: Amygdala and local anesthetic kindled seizures show differences in pharmacological responsivity as a function of kindling stage (++, very effective; ±, partially effective; 0, not effective). The double dissociation in response to diazepam and phenytoin in the early versus the late phases of amygdala kindling, as described by Pinel, is particularly striking. Note also that carbamazepine is effective in inhibiting the developmental phase of local anesthetic but not amygdala kindling, whereas the converse is true for the completed phase. ECS, electroconvulsant seizures.*

anticonvulsant substance in the kindling model. In both instances, TRH increases are driven by increases in gene transcription (i.e. there is a cellular signal that arrives at the nucleus which turns on the gene for TRH) (Figure 6.5) A messenger RNA (mRNA) is read off the DNA portion encoding TRH, and this mRNA for TRH then instructs the cell to synthesize more TRH peptide. It does this by stringing together, in the correct sequence, the appropriate amino acid building blocks that constitute the TRH peptide. Thus, transient increases in TRH and other anticonvulsant neuropeptides may help to try to re-establish equilibrium and prevent further seizures from occurring.

## Pathological vs adaptive changes in gene expression

In this way it is possible to conceptualize that the repeated occurrence of seizures in the kindling process or, by analogy, affective episodes, may not only be propelling the animal or human toward easier triggering of further episodes, but may also be engendering the body's own adaptations in attempts at preventing future episodes. However, these endogenous adaptations (such as TRH) tend to be relatively short-lived (Figure 6.9). As TRH peptide levels return to normal, the kindled animal or recurrent depressed patient (Figure 6.5) is again more highly vulnerable to recurrences (Figure 6.10). It is important to re-emphasize that kindling is not a literal model of affective disorder because motor seizures are not a manifestation of the illness. However, the development and regular occurrence of seizures in the amygdala kindling model, as well as their becoming spontaneous, provide an easily identifiable and studied endpoint. We can examine some of the general conceptual principles underlying this type of illness progression and ask whether they are pertinent to the affective disorders. This may be the case even if seizures and affective episodes are mediated via different neurochemical systems in the brain.

As noted above, in the different phases of kindling, there are very different neural substrates involved and a very different profile of effective pharmacology (Figure 6.7). Similarly, we believe that different stages of affective illness may also be differentially amenable to treatment interventions (Figure 6.10). In the kindling model, Dr Susan Weiss and

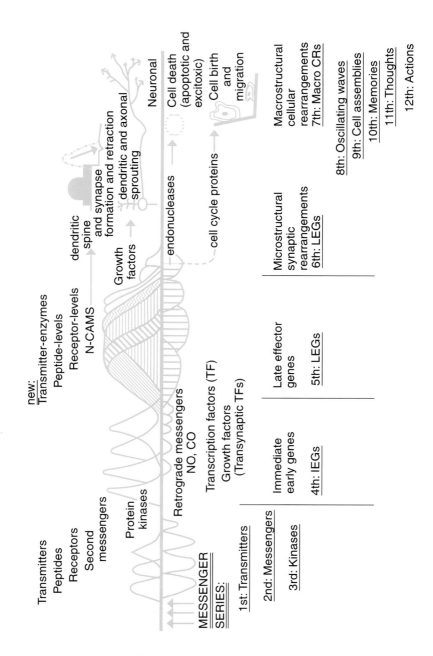

Transmitters
Peptides
Receptors
Second
messengers

new:
Transmitter-enzymes
Peptide-levels
Receptor-levels
N-CAMS

dendritic
spine
and synapse
formation and retraction

dendritic and axonal
sprouting

Cell death
(apoptotic and
excitoxic)

Neuronal

Cell birth
and
migration

Protein
kinases

Retrograde messengers
NO, CO

Growth
factors

endonucleases

cell cycle proteins

Transcription factors (TF)
Growth factors
(Transynaptic TFs)

MESSENGER
SERIES:

1st: Transmitters

2nd: Messengers

3rd: Kinases

4th: IEGs

Immediate
early genes

Late effector
genes

5th: LEGs

Microstructural
synaptic
rearrangements
6th: LEGs

Macrostructural
cellular
rearrangements
7th: Macro CRs

8th: Oscillating waves

9th: Cell assemblies

10th: Memories

11th: Thoughts

12th: Actions

colleagues have observed that animals treated with effective anticonvulsants earlier (compared with later) in the course of developing full-blown seizures are more likely to stay seizure free and are less likely to lose responsivity via a tolerance mechanism. Also, higher doses of drugs, stable rather than escalating doses, drugs with a higher initial degree of effectiveness, and combinations are more likely to remain effective than lower doses or use of marginally effective agents in monotherapy.

Some of these treatment principles for slowing the development of loss of efficacy (treatment resistance or tolerance) derived from the kindling model may be pertinent to affective disorders and re-emphasize the potential importance of early treatment with full doses of the best available drugs for sustained therapeutic effects. However, each of the predictions from the kindling model (Table 6.1) needs to be tested directly in the clinic for its ultimate applicability to patients. Nonetheless, they raise the issue as to whether early intervention with effective treatment at first onset of symptoms could prevent the entire syndrome from developing in a full-blown fashion. Whether the same drugs that are effective in the treatment of adult bipolar illness (Figure 6.10) are also effective in children and adolescents remains for further study. It is possible that with the highly plastic and changing neurochemistry of the nervous system, a different pharmacology will be required for the youngest children with the earliest affective illness manifestations.

---

*Figure 6.8* *Remodeling the central nervous system based on experience. This figure portrays an evolving cascade of messenger systems, each with its own complex regulatory mechanisms and crosstalk with other systems (not illustrated). In addition to showing immediate early genes (IEGs) and late effector genes (LEGs), this figure suggests that environmental stimulation can engage mechanisms that change the connectivity of the brain on a biochemical as well as microstructural basis, including cell sprouting, cell migration, or even cell death. These synaptic changes may ultimately be reflected in larger functional units (eighth and ninth messengers) that encode thoughts, memories, and preparation for action. NO, nitric oxide; CO, carbon monoxide; N-CAMS, neural cell adhesion molecules.*

Table 6.1 Clinical predictions[a] to be explored based on observations from a preclinical model of amygdala-kindled seizures[b]

| **Preclinical studies** | **Future studies; is there predictive validity for clinical tolerance in affective illness?** |
|---|---|
| *Tolerance to anticonvulsant effects is slowed by:* | *Would tolerance be slowed by?:* |
| a. Higher doses (except w/LTG) | a. Maximum tolerated doses |
| b. Not escalating doses | b. Stable dosing |
| c. More efficacious drugs (VPA > CBZ) | c. Different rate of treatment resistance (CBZ > VPA) |
| d. Treatments initiated early in illness | d. Early institution of lithium treatment is more effective than late |
| e. Combination treatment (CBZ + VPA) | e. Combination > monotherapy |
| f. Reducing illness drive | f. Treat co-morbidities |
| *Treatment response restored by:* | |
| a. Period of drug discontinuation then re-exposure | a. Randomized study of continuation treatment vs discontinuation and re-exposure needed |
| b. Agents with different mechanisms of action, i.e. no cross-tolerance (Cross tolerance from lamotrigine to CBZ, not VPA) | b. VPA should be more effective in those tolerant to LTG than to CBZ |

[a] Right side of table; [b] Left side of table

VPA, valproic acid; CBZ, carbamazepine; LTG, lamotrigine

## Implications for early intervention

It thus becomes a crucial question as to which agent to use to intervene most effectively in affective dysregulation of childhood and adolescence. Effective preventive treatment (pharmacoprophylaxis) would have many obvious benefits. Children would not only be saved from the considerable pain and suffering of mood swings and manic and depressive episodes (Figure 6.1), but also from their adverse social and educational consequences. Untreated bipolar illness often has a dramatic impact on friends, family, and schooling. The extent to which these factors can be lessened by appropriate pharmacotherapy would be of significance in its own right.

However, it is also possible (as the kindling and stress sensitization models predict) that effective early treatment intervention could prevent the increased vulnerability to subsequent recurrences, and actually change the predicted course of illness. Adolescents are recognized to be at risk for suicide with severe affective disorders and this is the population in which suicide is rising most rapidly. Moreover, the occurrence of bipolar illness appears to be a particularly high-risk factor for the subsequent development of alcohol and substance abuse. Because of these factors, juvenile and adolescent bipolar illness should be considered for early intervention, not only to attempt to prevent the development of full-blown affective episodes, but also to prevent many of the secondary adverse consequences of the illness.

It is highly promising that in adult bipolar illness there are now a multiplicity of treatment options (Figure 6.11). Unimodal antidepressants, antimanic, or antipsychotic agents as well as drugs like lithium have the ability to be effective in both manic and depressive phases, particularly in the prevention of recurrences. Which are the most effective mood stabilizers in children thus deserves the most careful clinical and research attention.

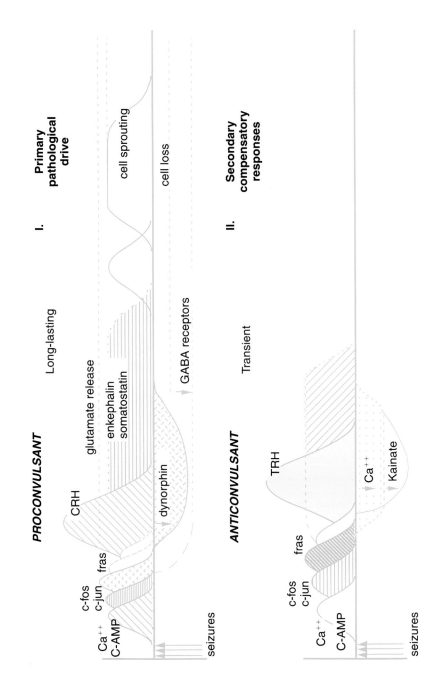

## Neurochemistry of affective illness

### Serotonin (5-HT)

Serotonin is one of a number of transmitters in cells that helps to convey electrical messages from one cell to the next across a synapse. That is, an electrical impulse releases chemical transmitters such as serotonin (5-HT) into the area (synapse) between cells, 5-HT binds to a receptor site on the second cell (the post-synaptic site), which then is associated with activation and firing of the second neuron. A deficiency of serotonin was postulated as a vulnerability factor in the development of recurrent affective illness (Coppen et al 1972) and in the increased impulsivity associated with suicide attempts and completed suicide.

The serotonin-permissive theory suggests that a relative deficiency of 5-HT can result in depression and also forms the basis for the mood overswings in mania caused by other factors. This theory has had much support with the development of serotonin-selective re-uptake inhibitor (SSRI) antidepressants, which increase serotonergic tone in the synapse by preventing the re-uptake or inactivation of serotonin, thus making 5-HT more available for a longer time to act on the post-synaptic receptors (Figure 6.12). Serotonergic mechanisms have most recently been clearly implicated in unipolar depression, with a tryptophan depletion test.

---

**Figure 6.9** *Schematic illustration of potential genomic, neurotransmitter, and peptidergic alterations that follow repeated kindled seizures. Putative mechanisms related to the primary pathological drive (i.e. kindled seizure evolution) are illustrated on top and those thought to be related to the secondary compensatory responses (i.e. anticonvulsant effects) are shown on the bottom. The horizontal line represents time. Sequential transient increases in second messengers and immediate effector genes (IEGs) are followed by longer lasting alterations in peptides, neurotransmitters, and receptors or their mRNAs, as illustrated above the line, whereas decreases are shown below the line. Given the potential unfolding of these competing mechanisms in the evolution of seizure disorders, the question arises regarding whether parallel opposing processes also occur in the course of affective illness or in other psychiatric disorders. Endogenous adaptive changes (bottom) may be exploited in the design of the new treatment strategies. TRH, thyrotropin-releasing hormone; Ca, calcium; C-AMP, cyclic adenosine monophosphate; GABA, gamma-aminobutryic acid; CRH, corticotropin-releasing hormone; fras, fos-related antigens.*

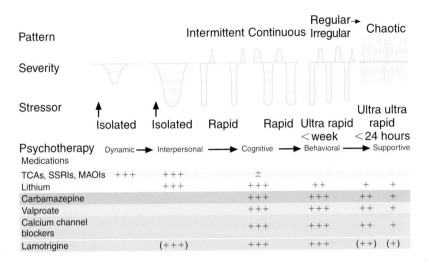

| Pattern | | Intermittent | Continuous | Regular→ Irregular | Chaotic |
|---|---|---|---|---|---|
| Severity | | | | | |
| Stressor | ↑ Isolated | ↑ Isolated | Rapid | Rapid Ultra rapid <week | Ultra ultra rapid <24 hours |
| Psychotherapy | Dynamic → | Interpersonal → | Cognitive → | Behavioral → | Supportive |
| Medications | | | | | |
| TCAs, SSRIs, MAOIs | +++ | +++ | ± | | |
| Lithium | | +++ | +++ | ++ | + + |
| Carbamazepine | | | +++ | +++ | ++ + |
| Valproate | | | +++ | +++ | ++ + |
| Calcium channel blockers | | | +++ | +++ | ++ + |
| Lamotrigine | | (+++) | +++ | +++ | (++) (+) |

*Figure 6.10* *Phases in the evolution of mood cycling; potential relationship to treatment response. In an analogous fashion to kindling, episodes of affective illness may progress from triggered (arrows) to spontaneous and show different patterns and frequencies (top) as a function of the stage of syndrome evolution. Just as different neural substrates are involved in different phases of kindling evolution, a similar principle is postulated in affective illness; these phases might also be responsive to different types of pharmacotherapies or psychotherapies. Although systematic and controlled studies have not examined the relationship of the illness phase to treatment response, anecdotal observations provide suggestive data that some treatments may be: differentially (+++) highly effective; (++) moderately effective; or (+) possibly effective, as a function of course of illness. Note that the pharmacological dissociations in the nonhomologous model of kindling are different from those postulated in mood disorders; nonetheless, the principle of differential response as a function of stage may be useful, and deserves to be specifically examined and tested. The use of multiple agents in combination as a function of late or severe illness stage is standard in many medical illnesses and should be studied systematically in the refractory mood disorders. TCAs, tricyclic antidepressants; SSRIs, serotonin-selective re-uptake inhibitors; MAOIs, monoamine oxidase inhibitors. Parentheses '( )' represent inconclusive evidence.*

When adult patients who have responded to an SSRI are given a diet of amino acids deficient in tryptophan (which is the precursor to serotonin), their mood is transiently worsened for a period of several hours, indicating that blocking serotonin production because of the deficiency of brain tryptophan transiently is associated with this lowering of mood.

**ANTIMANIC**

| | Typical neuroleptics | Atypical antipsychotics |
|---|---|---|
| High potency | Block D$_2$ receptors | Block mesolimbic Dopamine D$_1$, D$_2$, D$_4$ |
| Benzodiazepines | Chlorpromazine | receptors and 5HT$_2$ receptors |
| | Thioridazine | Clozapine, Olanzapine, Risperidone |
| ↑Cl⁻ influx | Haloperidol | Quetiapine, Ziprasidone, Aripiperazole |
| (Clonazepam, Lorazepam) | | |

**MOOD STABILIZERS**

| ↓2nd messenger | ↑GABA | ↓Glutamate | Dihydropyridine ↓Calcium | ↑Thyroid | ?Atypical antipsychotics |
|---|---|---|---|---|---|
| and G protein | Valproate | Carbamazepine | Nimodipine | | |
| Lithium | (Gabapentin*) | Lamotrigine | Isradipine | T$_3$ (25µg) | |
| Carbamazepine | (Tiagabine*) | Topiramate | (Amlodipine) | ↑↑T$_4$ (400–500µg) | |
| Valproate | | | | | |

**ANTIDEPRESSANTS**

| Dopamine | Serotonin (5HT) | 5HT plus | Norepinephrine (Ne) | 5HT and Ne | MAOI |
|---|---|---|---|---|---|
| Bupropion | Fluoxetine | Nefazodone | Desipramine | Clomipramine | Tranylcypromide |
| (Pramipexole) | Sertraline | Mirtazapine | Nortriptyline | Venlafaxine | Phenelzine |
| | Paroxetine | | Maprotiline | | Isocarboxazid |
| | Fluvoxamine | | Reboxitine | | [Moclobemide] |
| | Citalopram | | | | |

*Not antimanic or mood stabilizing

**Figure 6.11** Actions of antimanic agents, antidepressants, and mood stabilizers. Cl, Chloride; GABA, gamma-aminobutryic acid; T$_3$, triiodothyronine; T$_4$, levothyroxine; MAOI, monoamine oxidase inhibitors.

## Dopamine (DA) and norepinephrine (Ne)

Two other transmitters dopamine and norepinephrine, called catecholamines, are in different cells in the midbrain and brain stem and were also postulated by Schildkraut, Bunney, and Davis more than 30 years ago to be deficient in depression and excessive in mania (Figure 6.13). There is some evidence to support this viewpoint from the biochemical perspective and, in terms of mechanism of action of drugs, there is considerable support for such a theory. For example, the antipsychotic drugs (major tranquilizers or neuroleptics) that block the action of DA at the receptor are antimanic agents as well as the treatment of choice for the psychosis of schizophrenia (Figure 6.14). Moreover, blocking the synthesis of DA and Ne has also been associated with antimanic effects. Excesses in Ne in the spinal fluid of manic patients has also been found directly in adult manic patients studied on our clinical research unit.

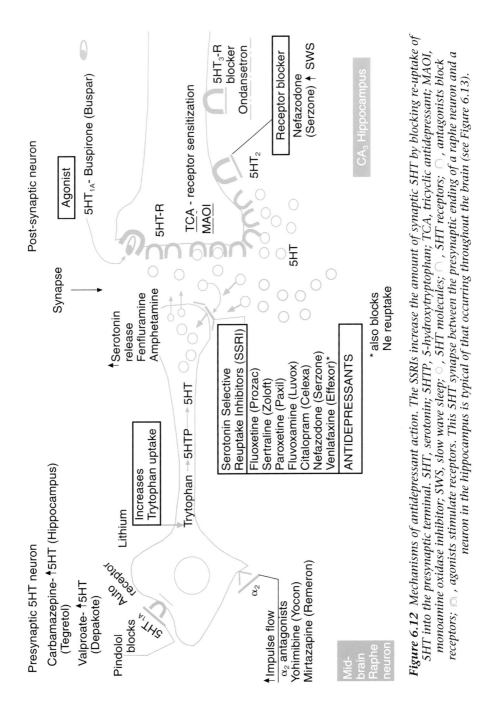

**Figure 6.12** *Mechanisms of antidepressant action. The SSRIs increase the amount of synaptic 5HT by blocking re-uptake of 5HT into the presynaptic terminal. 5HT, serotonin; 5HTP, 5-hydroxytryptophan; TCA, tricyclic antidepressant; MAOI, monoamine oxidase inhibitor; SWS, slow wave sleep; ○, 5HT molecules; ∩, 5HT receptors; ∩, antagonists block receptors; ◎, agonists stimulate receptors. This 5HT synapse between the presynaptic ending of a raphe neuron and a neuron in the hippocampus is typical of that occurring throughout the brain (see Figure 6.13).*

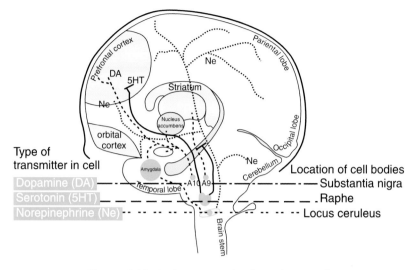

**Figure 6.13** *Amine systems implicated in mood.*

Neuroendocrine and peptide effects

Sachar and a number of other investigators demonstrated that depressed patients consistently secreted too much of the adrenal stress hormone cortisol during depressive episodes, and that this oversecretion normalized with recovery (Sachar et al 1973) If one gave a synthetic steroid such as dexamethasone to normal volunteers, this completely stopped cortisol production in the adrenal system because of the body's feedback messages that there were high levels of the circulating dexamethasone. However, approximately 50% of severely depressed patients given the same dose of dexamethasone that suppresses cortisol in normal volunteers failed to suppress cortisol. This has now become one of the most widely replicated findings in the clinical neuroscience of depression, and suggests that there is an increased drive in the hypo-thalamic–pituitary–adrenal axis (HPA) that controls cortisol secretion (Figure 6.15).

There is now direct evidence that corticotropin-releasing hormone (CRH) is hypersecreted in a subgroup of severely depressed patients, as measured indirectly in the spinal fluid of depressed patients in some but

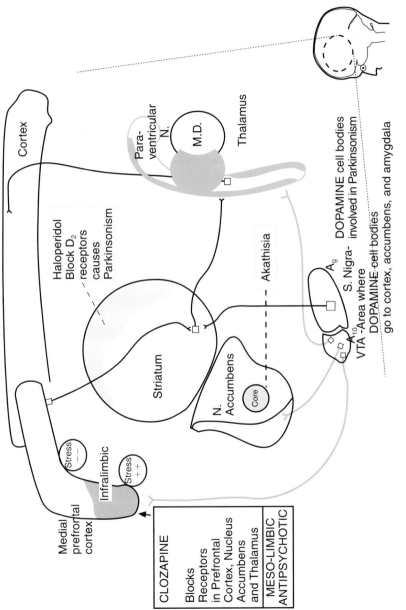

**Figure 6.14** *The atypical antipsychotic clozapine acts selectively on mesocortical dopamine (dark shading); the neuroleptic haloridol acts on the striatum and produces parkinsonism and on the core of the nucleus accumbens to produce akathisia (light shading). VTA, ventral segmental area; S. nigra, substantia nigra; M.D., mesocortical dopamine.*

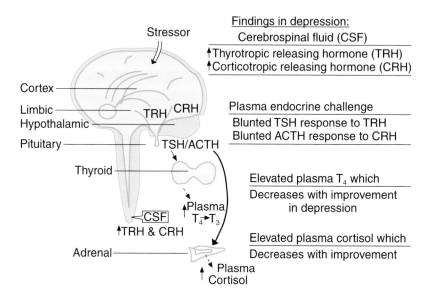

**Figure 6.15** *The corto-limbic HPA and HPT axis in depression. HPA, hypothalamic-pituitary adrenal; HPT, hypothalamic-pituitary-thyroid; ACTH, adrenocorticotropic hormone; $T_4$, levothyroxine; $T_3$, triiodothyronine; TSH, thyroid-stimulating hormone.*

not all studies. Thus, an increased amount of CRH in the hypothalamus would increase adrenocorticotropic hormone (ACTH) secretion from the pituitary and release cortisol from the adrenal. When this happens in Cushing's disease, the hypercortisolemia is associated with fatigue, cognitive impairment, and depression in a high percentage of patients.

In a similar manner, the functional endocrine disturbance of depression is thought, at least in part, to be related to such hypercortisolemia driven by increases in CRH. It is worth noting that many of the effective antidepressant agents do, in fact, exert mechanisms that reverse this hypersecretion of cortisol. Failure to normalize the dexamethasone suppression test or the CRH hyperactivity is associated with an increased risk of relapse.

In addition to CRH, in depressive illness there is also evidence of increased secretion of thyrotropin-releasing hormone (TRH), another peptide localized in the hypothalamus, that releases thyroid-stimulating hormone (TSH) from the pituitary and allows the thyroid gland to release $T_4$ as well as $T_3$. Depressed patients also tend to hypersecrete these thyroid hormones, which normalizes with improvement in the depression. Such hypersecretion is evidenced by a blunted TSH response to an intravenous injection of TRH (presumably because the TSH receptor is downregulated secondary to the TRH excesses).

In contrast to CRH, which is thought to be intimately involved in the symptoms of depression, TRH hypersecretion (Figures 6.5 and 6.9) may represent one of a number of the body's compensatory mechanisms that attempt to restabilize the patient and act as an internal (or endogenous) antidepressant. We think that this is the case because studies using intravenous TRH have suggested that it has antidepressant effects (Prange Jr et al 1972). Moreover, when we directly injected TRH into patients' spinal fluid in order to allow sufficient quantities to reach the brain, we found that TRH had antidepressant, antianxiety, and antisuicidal effects in a small group of highly treatment-refractory patients studied at the NIMH (Callahan et al 1997; Marangell et al 1997).

Thus, because these two peptides (CRH as a representative of an endogenous 'bad guy' and TRH as a representative of an endogenous 'good guy') with apparently opposite effects on depression are both hypersecreted during episodes, it is thought that their relative ratio might account for the periods of illness or well intervals between episodes (Figure 6.5). That is, when CRH and other pathological factors are hypersecreted out of proportion to compensatory mechanisms, depression occurs. However, when the adaptive factors typified by TRH predominate, periods of 'wellness' may emerge (Post and Weiss 1992).

This formulation not only helps to conceptualize why the illness may fluctuate with periods of illness and recovery between episodes, but it also provides a new set of targets for therapeutics. Not only would one want to inhibit the 'bad guys' (CRH and cortisol hypersecretion), but also to enhance the 'good guys' (such as TRH and certain other alterations associated with an affective episode that may be helpful in ending it). Some effort in this direction of boosting TRH is being pursued by Dr Winokur and associates at the University of Connecticut.

There is also evidence that the peptide somatostatin (SRIF) (Figure 6.5) is decreased during periods of depression and returns to normal with recovery (Rubinow et al 1987). This is of considerable interest because somatostatin is decreased in the brains of patients with Alzheimer's disease in proportion to the severity of cognitive impairment. Thus, it is possible that some of the cognitive difficulties that depressed patients transiently experience could be related to alterations in this and other critical chemicals involved in normal cognition, learning and memory, such as DA and Ne. However, in contrast to Alzheimer's disease in which cells are permanently damaged or gone, the deficit in gene expression of somatostatin in depression is temporary and normalizes when the patient recovers.

## Intracellular ions

Another highly consistent finding in depression is increased intracellular calcium in blood elements of affectvely ill patients compared with healthy volunteers. The precise mechanism of this alteration is not known, but it is hoped that its identification in peripheral cells, i.e. those circulating in blood, might lead to the identification of similar mechanisms that could be involved in parallel in the increased intracellular calcium in brain cells (neurons). There is some evidence that the defect in intracellular calcium is a marker for the illness, since it has been identified in cultured cells from bipolar patients that have undergone immortalization and multiple replications.

Thus, it would appear that there is something inherent in the genetics of the cells rather than the biochemical milieu in which they circulate that accounts for such calcium increases. These data are also of interest in relation to the recent finding that a variety of agents effective in the treatment of affective illness appear to exert effects on blocking calcium influx into neurons in the brain, and these agents include not only the direct voltage-sensitive calcium channel blockers of the dihydropyridine class, such as nimodipine, isradipine, and amlodipine, but also mood-stabilizing agents, such as lithium, carbamazepine, valproate, and lamotrigine, which slow calcium influx through the $N$-methyl-D-aspartate (NMDA)-type glutamate receptor.

## The effect of lithium carbonate on intracellular messengers and neurotrophic factors

With the recognition that the lithium ion was effective in the treatment of bipolar illness it was hoped that an understanding of its mechanism of action would rapidly lead to a clarification of the pathological mechanisms involved in the illness (Figure 6.16). Unfortunately, this has not proven to be easy because lithium has a multiplicity of biochemical effects, and which of these is most important to its effects on mood has not been adequately defined. In addition, the absence of a suitable animal model for manic-depressive illness has clearly hampered such an investigative route. With a variety of mood-stabilizing anticonvulsants now available, such as carbamazepine, valproate, and perhaps a second generation of agents such as lamotrigine and topiramate, one can further hope to identify convergent mechanisms of action. Thus, finding common mechanisms among the mood stabilizers may aid in the uncovering of the biochemical alterations involved in the illness.

Dr H. Manji has used this process as the basis for treating animals chronically with lithium and valproate in the hope of identifying common biochemical alterations that occur with these two agents, and looking for commonalities among these two different chemical substances (an ion and a fatty acid) that might provide new clues. They found that lithium and valproate shared a number of actions in common, one of which was the inhibition of a critical intracellular enzyme or second messenger called protein kinase C (PKC) (Manji et al 1996).

They went on to test the hypothesis that inhibition of this enzyme might be associated with therapeutic actions by using a PKC inhibitor (tamoxifen) that had already been approved for use in other illnesses. Tamoxifen, in addition to its effects at the estrogen receptor that make it useful in the treatment of breast cancer, is also a highly potent PKC inhibitor. Manji and colleagues thus used tamoxifen in acute manic patients and found rapid onset effects in six of the first seven manic patients treated (Bebchuk et al 2000). These investigators hope to test a more specific PKC inhibitor that does not share the estrogenic effects of tamoxifen to further clarify such a potential new target of therapeutics.

In addition to the PKC mechanisms, lithium and valproate also affect

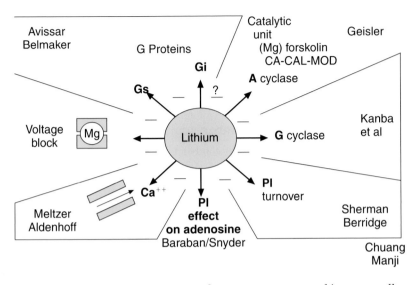

**Figure 6.16** *Lithium acts on second messenger systems and increases cell survival factors and decreases cell death factors. Mg, magnesium; Ca, calcium; PI, phospoinositol; A, adenylate.*

a variety of intracellular second and third messenger systems including effects on G-proteins (the mechanism that links receptor activation to intracellular processes and calcium). Both of these drugs also increase binding at a specific site on DNA called activator protein-1 (AP-1). AP-1 changes gene transcription. It is thought that these effects might be associated with the ability of lithium to increase brain-derived neurotrophic factor (BDNF) and also the neuroprotective protein Bcl-2 that prevents cells from undergoing preprogrammed cell death or apoptosis, i.e. a form of cell suicide. Dr Chuang and colleagues in our laboratory also found that lithium inhibited cell death factors (BAX and p53) and that it increased survival of neurons in culture and in animal models of stroke and Huntington's disease. These effects could be important in humans because lithium now appears to increase a marker of neuronal integrity, *N*-acetyl aspartate (NAA) and the amount of grey matter in humans, as measured by new brain imaging techniques. Whether these actions are critical to lithium's therapeutic effects in bipolar illness remains to be demonstrated.

## Physiology and biochemistry of depression

### Brain imaging and autopsy studies

Dramatic new technical developments have allowed the examination of functional brain activity in an awake, behaving individual. Positron emission tomography (PET) can measure metabolism with 18-fluorodeoxyglucose or blood flow with oxygen-15 water and convey precise information about regional brain activity during depression, mania, and normal states.

A large number of studies have indicated that depressed patients have decrements in activity (either blood flow or metabolism) in the frontal cortex (Figure 6.17, Post 2000), often in proportion to the severity of depression as rated on the Hamilton depression scale. In many instances this deficit is reported to normalize on recovery from depression. However, in the case of treatment with electroconvulsive therapy, Sackeim and colleagues have found that successful treatment appears to be associated with further decrements in the frontal hypoactivity rather than its normalization.

There is also considerable evidence linking affective illness to alterations in the size and activity of structures in the medial part of the temporal lobe or limbic system, such as the amygdala, hippocampus, and parahippocampal gyrus, that are thought to be intimately involved in modulation of emotion and cognition. Thus, these modern brain imaging techniques are beginning to provide confirmatory evidence of limbic dysfunction that has long been postulated based on indirect data from humans or in laboratory studies of emotion in animals.

Papez (1937) first suggested that the limbic circuit was associated with modulation of emotion and this concept has been advanced further by MacLean (1973) and many others. If this part of the brain is stimulated directly with depth electrodes in patients with epilepsy, a variety of emotional and experiential phenomena are induced, including considerable degrees of anxiety.

Dr Ketter in our group has shown that the local anesthetic procaine is a relatively selective activator of the amygdala and its outflow pathways into the insula, anterior cingulate gyrus, and orbital frontal cortex. The

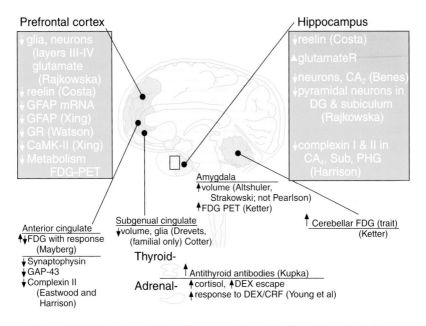

**Figure 6.17** *Bipolar affective illness: anatomy, biochemistry, physiology. GFAP, glial fibrillary acidic protein; CaMK-II, calcium calmodulin kinase-II; FDG, flourodeoxyglucose; PET, positron emission tomography; DEX, dexamethasone; CRF, corticotropin-releasing factor; Sub, subiculum; PHG, parahippocampal gyrus; DG, dentate gyrus.*

infusion of procaine is associated with either euphoric or dysphoric affects, further supporting the concept of limbic modulation of emotional function. Depressed patients have altered responsivity to procaine, with a decreased response in these crucial areas of the brain (Ketter et al 1996).

An increase in the size of the amygdala in bipolar illness has been reported by a number of investigators (Brambilla et al 2001). Decreases in the number and activity of glial cells have been found in the frontal cortex and related areas of the brain, such as the anterior cingulate gyrus, by several investigators (Rajkowska 2000). Guoqiang Xing in our laboratory has found the enzyme, calcium calmodulin kinase-IIα (CaMK-IIα), which responds to calcium signals and is necessary for long-term memory, is decreased in the frontal cortex of those who had manic-depressive illness compared with controls (Xing et al 2002). Such a deficit, along with other changes, could account for some of the difficulties in cognition experienced by our patients. There are data suggesting that alterations in the hippocampus and anterior cingulate occur in proportion to the duration of the illness, and in the size of the third ventricle (in proportion to the degree of cognitive deficit).

## Neurological and psychiatric overlaps

We are beginning to have an understanding of some of the alterations in physiology and biochemistry that accompany major fluctuations in mood. The data on genetics and the very well-replicated findings of peptide, endocrine, and calcium alterations in bipolar illness and the consistent deficits in prefrontal cortex activity and biochemistry (Figure 6.17) place depression very much in the realm of other medical disorders with not only distinct mood, motor, and vegetative symptoms, but also an increasingly well-delineated neurobiology.

While the 'functional' or reversible brain lesions of psychiatry have often been referred to as somehow less robust or less well documented than those of neurology (such as stroke, tumors, or neural degeneration), the information on the fundamental neurobiology of the affective disorders is beginning to alter this perspective and to place the affective illnesses and schizophrenia in the realm of true brain disorders. In fact the functional nature of these illnesses suggests that they may be somewhat more difficult to understand but much more amenable to treatment and therefore equally deserving of considerable research efforts and novel attempts at clinical therapeutics. This is even more true because the affective illnesses are potentially lethal medical disorders with a lifetime incidence rate of suicide between 10 and 20%. Long-term treatment with lithium tends to normalize the suicide rate toward that of the general population, raising the hope that treatment with this agent and others will eventually help ameliorate not only the morbidity but also the mortality of the affective disorders.

## Further reading

Bebchuk JM, Arfken CL, Dolan-Manji S et al (2000) A preliminary investigation of a protein kinase C inhibitor in the treatment of acute mania. *Arch Gen Psychiatry* **57**:95–7.

Berrettini WH, Ferraro TN, Goldin LR et al (1994) Chromosome 18 DNA markers and manic-depressive illness: evidence for a susceptibility gene. *Proc Natl Acad Sci USA* **91**:5918–21.

Biederman J, Faraone S, Mick E et al (1996) Attention-deficit hyperactivity disorder and juvenile mania: an overlooked comorbidity? *J Am Acad Child Adolesc Psychiatry* **35**:997–1008.

Brambilla P, Harenski K, Nicoletti ME et al (2001) Are amygdala volumes increased in bipolar disorder patients? *Bipolar Disorders* **3**:28.

Callahan AM, Frye MA, Marangell LBT et al (1997) Comparative antidepressant effects of intravenous and intrathecal thyrotropin-releasing hormone: confounding effects of tolerance and implications for therapeutics. *Biol Psychiatry* **41**:264–72.

Coppen A, Prange AJ Jr, Whybrow PC et al (1972) Abnormalities of indoleamines in affective disorders. *Arch Gen Psychiatry* **26**:474–8.

Craddock N, Jones I (1999): Genetics of bipolar disorder. *J Med Genet* **36**: 585–94.

Gershon ES, Hamovit JH, Guroff J, Nurnberger JI (1987) Birth-cohort changes in manic and depressive disorders in relatives of bipolar and schizoaffective patients. *Arch Gen Psychiatry* **44**:314–19.

Kessing LV, Andersen PK, Mortensen PB et al (1998) Recurrence in affective disorder. I. Case register study. *Br J Psychiatry* **172**:23–8.

Ketter TA, Andreason PJ, George MS et al (1996) Anterior paralimbic mediation of procaine-induced emotional and psychosensory experiences. *Arch Gen Psychiatry* **53**:59–69.

Kraepelin E (1921) *Manic-depressive insanity and paranoia.* (Robertson GM, ed., trans. Barclay RM) Edinburgh: Livingstone.

Lange KJ and McInnis MG (2002) Studies of anticipation in bipolar affective disorder. *CNS Spectrums* **7**:196–202.

Leverich GS, McElroy SL, Suppes T et al (2001) Early physical or sexual abuse and the course of bipolar illness. *Biol Psychiatry* **51**:288–97.

Li R, el Mallakh RS (1997) Triplet repeat gene sequences in neuropsychiatric diseases. *Harv Rev Psychiatry* **5**:66–74.

MacLean PD (1973) A triune concept of the brain and behavior. In The Clarence M. Hicks memorial lectures (eds Boag TJ, Campbell D) 1969. Toronto: University of Toronto Press.

Manji HK, Bersudsky, Y, Chen G et al (1996) Modulation of protein kinase C isozymes and substrates by lithium: the role of myo-inositol. *Neuropsychopharmacology* **15**:370–81.

Marangell LB, George MS, Callahan AM et al (1997) Effects of intrathecal thyrotropin-releasing hormone (protirelin) in refractory depressed patients. *Arch Gen Psychiatry* **54**:214–22.

McMahon FJ, Hopkins PJ, Xu J et al (1997) Linkage of bipolar affective disorder to chromosome 18 markers in a new pedigree series. *Am J Hum Genet* **61**: 1397–404.

Mendlewicz J, Lindbald K, Souery D et al (1997) Expanded trinucleotide CAG repeats in families with bipolar affective disorder. *Biol Psychiatry* **42**:1115–22.

Papez, JW (1937) A proposed mechanism of emotion. *Arch Neurol Psychiatry* **38**: 725–43.

Post RM (1992) Transduction of psychosocial stress into the neurobiology of recurrent affective disorder. *Am J Psych* **149**:999–1010.

Post RM, Weiss SR (1992) Ziskind-Somerfeld Research Award 1992. Endogenous biochemical abnormalities in affective illness: therapeutic versus pathogenic. *Biol Psychiatry* **32**:469–84.

Post RM (2000) Neural substrates of psychiatric syndromes. In Principles of Behavioral and Cognitive Neurology, 2nd edn (ed. Mesulam MM) New York: Oxford University Press, pp 406–38.

Prange AJ Jr, Lara PP, Wilson IC et al (1972) Effects of thyrotropin-releasing hormone in depression. *Lancet* **11**:999–1002.

Rajkowska G (2000) Postmortem studies in mood disorders indicate altered numbers of neurons and glial cells. *Biol Psychiatry* **48**:766–77.

Rubinow DR, Post RM, Davis C et al (1987) Somatostatin and depression. In *Somatostatin* (ed. Reichlin S) New York: Plenum Publishing, pp 183–92.

Sachar EJ, Hellman L, Roffwarg HP et al (1973) Disrupted 24-hour patterns of cortisol secretion in psychotic depression. *Arch Gen Psychiatry* **28**:19–24.

Stine OC, Xu J, Koskela R et al (1995) Evidence for linkage of bipolar disorder to chromosome 18 with a parent-of-origin effect. *Am J Hum Genet* **57**:1384–94.

Xing GQ, Russell S, Hough C et al (2002) Decreased prefrontal CaMKII α mRNA in bipolar illness. *Neuro Report* **13**:501–5.

# chapter 7

# Mood stabilizers

## Introduction

Current clinical practice is to treat manic episodes in children and adolescents with bipolar disorders (BPD) much as one would adults with these disorders, using mood stabilizers and antipsychotic agents (Hirschfeld 1994; Kafantaris 1995; McClellan and Werry 1997). With the increasing use of mood-stabilizing agents like lithium and valproate in children and adolescents with BPD, it is important to understand the risks and benefits of these agents and the literature supporting their use. Although there are emerging studies about the use of these agents in bipolar children and adolescents, there is still a paucity of controlled trials in this population. It is important to be familiar with the relevant adult BPD treatment literature as many times one is forced to generalize from these data to children and adolescents.

## Lithium

### Evidence for lithium

Lithium is the oldest and most well-studied mood stabilizer for adults with bipolar disorder. In the USA the Food and Drug Administration (FDA) approved lithium to be marketed for the treatment of manic episodes of BPD in 1970. Lithium has multiple, complex effects in the brain, particularly at the second messenger level that include blocking the activity of inositol polyphosphatase 1-phosphatase and inosito second messenger systems and inhibiting adenyl cyclase by competing with magnesium in this second messenger system (Cade 1949; Alessi, Naylor, Ghaziuddin et al 1994). New data suggest it may also have neurotropic and neuroprotective effects (Chuang et al 2002).

Five well-controlled studies have demonstrated that lithium is superior to placebo in the treatment of adults with acute mania (McElroy and Keck 2000). There have been five controlled trials of lithium in bipolar children and adolescents. Of these five studies, four (Gram and Rafaelsen 1972; Lena 1979; McKnew et al 1981; Delong and Nieman 1983) used a crossover design which has potential confounds for an illness that is cyclic in nature. The average number of subjects in each of these studies was 18 and response rates ranged from 33 to 80%. In the only well-controlled, prospective study, which utilized current DSM-IV diagnostic criteria for BPD, Geller and colleagues, administered lithium in a double-blinded and placebo-controlled fashion to 25 adolescents with a bipolar disorder and a secondary substance dependency disorder (most had alcohol and marijuana dependence) (Geller et al 1998). In this study, the adolescents' diagnosis of BPD preceded their substance abuse by several years. After 6 weeks of treatment, those subjects treated with lithium showed a significant decrease in their substance abuse and a significant improvement in their global assessment of functioning. This was the first well-controlled trial that clearly demonstrated the efficacy of lithium carbonate in the treatment of bipolar adolescents with comorbid substance abuse.

## Clinical use

Lithium is readily absorbed from the gastrointestinal system with peak levels occurring 2–4 hours after each dose. The kidneys excrete lithium and its serum half-life in children and adolescents is estimated to be approximately 18 hours (Vitiello et al 1988). Weller et al devised a lithium dosage guide for children and adolescents based upon body weight that is useful, accurate and easy to use with outpatients (Weller, Weller and Fristad 1986). According to these guidelines, in a 6–12-year-old child, a dose of 30 mg/kg/day in three divided doses will produce a lithium level of 0.6–1.2 mEq/l within five days. Lithium is usually administered 2–3 times/day and, after an adequate serum level is reached, in children it may be administered once in the morning and once at bedtime in a controlled release preparation. Serum lithium levels in the range 1.0–1.2 mEq/l are oftentimes necessary for mood stabilization during treatment of a child or adolescents during a manic episode and it is best to measure serum lithium levels 12 hours after the last dose. Initial therapeutic effects are usually seen within 10–14 days of achieving an adequate serum level, but full efficacy with lithium may not been seen for 4–6 weeks.

Lithium is available in the USA as tablets, capsules, two long-acting preparations (Eskalith and Lithobid), and as a liquid (lithium citrate). Caution should be used when switching a child from the tablet or long-acting preparation forms to lithium citrate as there is a report of an increase in serum lithium levels following a switch from the tablet to the liquid form of lithium (Reischer and Pfeffer 1996). Baseline studies prior to initiating treatment with lithium should include: general medical history and physical examination; serum electrolytes; creatinine, BUN, and serum calcium levels; thyroid function tests; ECG; complete blood count with differential; and a pregnancy test for sexually active females. Renal function should be tested every two to three months during the first six months of treatment with lithium carbonate, and thyroid function should be tested during the first six months of treatment. Thereafter, renal and thyroid functions should be checked every six months or when clinically indicated. Chronic treatment with lithium can potentially cause hyperparathyroidism so serum calcium levels should be checked at least once a year (Bendz et al 1996b).

Possible common side-effects of lithium in children and adolescents include nausea, diarrhea, acne, abdominal distress, sedation, tremor, polydypsia, polyuria, and weight gain. The long-term effects of lithium upon renal function in children and adolescents are not known, but in adults these effects have been found to be clinically insignificant but renal function should be monitored carefully in patients who are treated with lithium chronically (Bendz et al 1994; 1996a).

The therapeutic range for lithium is very narrow, 0.8–1.2 mEq/l, and lithium toxicity can occur at serum levels of 1.5 mEq/l or less. Signs and symptoms of lithium toxicity include tremor, blurred vision, nausea and diarrhea, ataxia, hyperreflexia, and dysarthria. During the hot summer months, children and adolescents should be told to drink plenty of fluids and their caretakers advised to contact the prescribing physician if signs of lithium toxicity occur.

Drug interactions with lithium are common and patients should be advised not to take any other medications without first consulting with their prescribing physician. The following medications may increase serum lithium levels: antibiotics (e.g. ampicillin and tetracycline), nonsteroidal anti-inflammatories (e.g. ibuprofen), antipsychotic agents, propanolol, and serotonin-selective re-uptake inhibitors (e.g. fluoxetine) (Ciraulo et al 1995). Lithium should be administered cautiously and serum levels monitored carefully in patients with significant renal, cardiovascular, or thyroid disease, or severe dehydration. Adequate birth control measures must be followed in adolescent females taking lithium, as lithium is associated with an increased rate of fetal cardiac abnormalities (Cohen et al 1994).

## Valproate

Valproate is a simple branched-chain carboxylic acid that was first introduced in the USA in 1978 as an anticonvulsant agent (Rimmer and Richens 1985). It is currently approved by the FDA to be marketed for the treatment of partial-complex seizures, migraines, and manic episodes of manic-depressive illness in adults. Valproate's exact mechanism of action in both seizure and mood disorders is unclear but appears to involve increased turnover of the inhibitory neurotransmitter GABA with potentiation of GABAergic functions, blockage of sodium channels and associated inhibition of glutamate release and attenuation of protein kinase C isoenzymes (Loscher 1993; Manji et al 1996).

### Evidence for valproate

A review of the five adult controlled valproate studies for the acute treatment of mania showed an average response rate of 54% (McElroy and Keck 2000). In many of these studies, positive results were obtained even though patients were selected from a population previously refractory to lithium treatment and those characterized by rapid cycling, mixed affective states, and irritability. There have been a number of older case reports and open prospective trials of valproate in bipolar children and adolescents that have suggested that it may be effective (Papatheodorou and Kutcher 1993; West et al 1994; Papatheodorou et al 1995; West 1995; Deltito et al 1998).

Recently, three prospective trials have also suggested that valproate may be effective in children and adolescents with pediatric BPD. Kowatch et al (2000) compared the efficacy of three mood stabilizers, lithium, valproate, and carbamazepine (CBZ), in the acute phase treatment of bipolar I or II children and adolescents during a mixed or manic episode. Subjects had to be medically healthy and have a normal intelligence. Excluded were those with current or lifetime diagnoses of schizophrenia, OCD, or autistic disorder; substance dependence or abuse; organic brain disease; and current use of psychotropic agents. In this study, 42 outpatients with a mean age of 11.4 years, were randomly assigned to 6–8 weeks of open treatment with lithium, valproate or CBZ; 20 patients met DSM-IV criteria for bipolar I disorder and 22 for bipolar II disorder, all with a mixed or manic episode. Patients' mean CGAS score was 48. Patients were stratified based on age, gender, and the presence of ADHD. The primary efficacy measures were the weekly Clinical Global Impression (CGI) improvement score and the Young Mania Rating Scale (Y-MRS). Using a $\geq 50\%$ change from baseline to exit in the Y-MRS scores to define response, the response rates were: CBZ 38%; lithium 38%; and sodium divalproex 53%. All three mood stabilizers were well tolerated and no serious adverse effects were seen.

Wagner et al (2001) have recently presented their results from an open-label study of valproate in 40 children and adolescents (aged 7–19 years) with a primary diagnosis of BPD. This study attempted to follow an open/discontinuation design in which all the patients were started on medication and were then randomized to either placebo or to medication when they improved, but too few subjects participated in the double-blind period to allow for statistical analysis of efficacy. In their initial open-label phase, subjects were given a starting dosage of valproate of 15 mg/kg/day. The mean final dosage was 17 mg/kg/day. Twenty-two subjects (55%) showed a 50% or more improvement in MRS scores during the open phase of treatment. Wagner and colleagues concluded that the study provided 'preliminary support for efficacy and safety of valproate in the treatment of bipolar disorder in children and adolescents'.

Delbello et al (2001) have recently published the results of the first, double-blind and placebo-controlled study that examined the efficacy, safety, and tolerability of quetiapine as an adjunct to valproate for acute mania in adolescents with BPD. In this study, 30 manic or mixed bipolar I adolescent inpatients, aged 12–18 years, received an initial valproate dose of 20 mg/kg and were randomized to 6 weeks of quetiapine with valpraote, which was titrated to 450 mg/day ($n = 15$), or valpraote and placebo ($n = 15$). The primary efficacy measures were change from baseline to endpoint in Y-MRS score and Y-MRS response rate. The valproate group demonstrated a 53% response rate whereas the valproate + quetiapine group demonstrated an 87% response rate. Table 7.1 summarizes the pediatric literature that suggests that valproate may be effective in treating adolescents during the acute manic phase of BPD. These results reveal a mean response rate of 54% to valproate in BPD children and adolescents. This response rate is based on only three studies, but the results were very consistent among the three.

## Clinical use

Valproate is readily absorbed from the gastrointestinal system with peak levels occurring 2–4 hours after each dose. However, if valproate is given with meals to decrease nausea, then peak levels may be reached in 5–6 hours. Valproate is highly protein bound, metabolized in the liver and has a serum half-life of 8–16 hours in children and young adolescents (Cloyd et al 1993). A starting dose of valproate of 15 mg/kg/day in 2–3 divided doses in children and adolescents will produce serum valproate levels in the range 50–60 mg/ml. Once this low serum level has been obtained, the dose is usually titrated upwards

Table 7.1  Valproate studies in child and adolescent bipolar disorders

| Study | Design | n | Mean age (years) | Trial duration (days) | Primary efficacy measure | Response rate by intent-to-treat sample |
|---|---|---|---|---|---|---|
| (Kowatch et al 2000) | Random, open, parallel group: lithium, DVP or CBZ | 42 | 11 | 42 | > 50% change from baseline in Y-MRS | DVP 53% |
| (Wagner et al 2001) | Open, prospect., mono-therapy with DVP | 40 | 11 | 56 | > 50% change from baseline in Y-MRS | DVP 55% |
| (DelBello et al 2002) | Random, parallel group: DVP + placebo or quetiapine + DVP | 30 | 14 | 42 | > 50% Change from baseline in Y-MRS | DVP 53% |

depending upon the subject's tolerance and response and it is best to measure serum valproate levels 8–12 hours after the last dose. Optimum serum levels among bipolar adults with mania appear to be 85–110 mg/ml and the same is probably true in bipolar children and adolescents (Bowden 1996). The maximum recommended daily dose of valproate is 60 mg/kg.

Baseline studies prior to initiating treatment with valproate should include: general medical history and physical examination; liver function tests; complete blood count with differential and platelets; and a pregnancy test for sexually active females. Complete blood count with differential, platelet count, and liver functions should be checked every six months or when clinically indicated. Possible common side-effects of valproate in children and adolescents include nausea, increased appetite, weight gain, sedation, thrombocytopenia, transient hair loss, tremor, and vomiting. Valproate is metabolized in the liver by the cytochrome P-450 system and has interactions with a number of other medications, which are also metabolized by this system. Medications that will increase valproate levels include: erythromycin, SSRIs, cimetidine, and salicylates. Valproate may increase the levels of the following medications: phenobarbital, primidone, carbamazepine, phenytoin, tricyclics, and notably lamotrigene (Ciraulo et al 1995). Valproate should be administered cautiously and serum levels and liver functions monitored carefully in patients with significant liver dysfunction. Adequate birth control measures must be followed in adolescent females taking valproate since it is associated with an increased rate of neural tube defects (Nau et al 1991).

There have been several reports in the neurology literature of valproate's association with a syndrome of obesity, hyperandrogenism, and polycystic ovaries in female patients treated for seizure disorders with valproate (Isojarvi et al 1993). Isojarvi has speculated that the cause of these valproate-related endocrine disorders seems to be from the valproate-induced obesity, which causes hypoinsulinemia, low serum levels of insulin-like growth factor-binding protein 1 and increases in serum sex hormones (Isojarvi et al 1996). However, more recent data from Rasgon and others indicate the syndrome of polycystic ovaries may be related to having epilepsy and not occur in females with BPD (Rasgon et al 2000; Luef et al 2001).

## Carbamazepine and oxcarbazepine

Carbamazepine, structurally similar to imipramine, is an anticonvulsant agent that was first introduced in the USA for the treatment of neuralgia in 1968. It is approved by the FDA to be marketed for the treatment of partial seizures with complex symptomatology, generalized tonic–clonic seizures, mixed seizure, and trigeminal neuralgia. Oxcarbazepine (Trileptal®) is the 10-keto analogue of carbamazepine, which has a distinct pharmacokinetic profile. In contrast to the oxidative metabolism of carbamazepine, oxcarbazepine is rapidly reduced to its active monohydroxy metabolite (Keck et al 1992). With the possible exception of the P-450IIIA isozyme of the P-450 family, neither oxcarbazepine nor its monohydroxy derivative induce hepatic oxidative metabolism. The primary pharmacological activity of oxcarbazepine is attributed to its 10-monohydroxy metabolite (MHD) because of the rapid systemic metabolism of the parent compound. Like most anticonvulsants, the exact mechanism of action is unknown; however, in vitro studies indicate that voltage-sensitive sodium channels are blocked, thereby stabilizing neural membranes, inhibiting repetitive neuronal firing, and diminishing synaptic impulse activity. Modulation of potassium and calcium channels may also be involved. GABA receptors are not affected by oxcarbazepine or MHD.

### Evidence for carbamazepine and oxcarbazepine

Carbamazepine has been found to be effective as a second-line treatment of acute mania in adults (Janicak et al 1997) but has never been studied in a controlled manner with bipolar children and adolescents. The majority of carbamazepine reports in the literature are with children and adolescents with attention-deficit/hyperactivity disorder (ADHD) or conduct disorder, some of whom also had neurological disorders (Puente 1975; Evans et al 1987; Kafantaris, et al 1992; Cueva et al 1996). Nine-

teen clinical trials have been completed using carbamazepine oxcarbazepine in adult bipolar patients and summarized by various investigators (Post et al 1996). Of these controlled or partially controlled studies,
64 patients were exposed to oxcarbazepine and compared to haloperidol, lithium or placebo. In most patients either better or comparable efficacy was observed with an average decrease in side-effects. In addition,
oxcarbazepine has been evaluated for efficacy in two double-blind clinical trials including a total of 96 patients (Emrich et al 1985). The control
drug was haloperidol in one trial, and lithium in the other; a placebo
control has not been used. Similar percentages of all treatment groups
improved. However, the frequent use of rescue medication throughout
the whole trial period makes precise comparisons difficult.

## Clinical use

Carbamazepine tends to be fairly sedating in children and because of
this adverse effect, and its many drug interactions, it is typically used as
an augmenting agent with lithium in those patients who do not respond
to lithium, valproate, or the combination of lithium and valproate. In
patients aged 6–12 years, a reasonable starting dose of carbamazepine is
100 mg twice daily and in patients aged 12 and older, 300 mg at night.
Serum levels of carbamazepine of 4–12 mg/ml are used for seizure
control. The maximum daily dose of carbamazepine should not exceed
1000 mg/day in children aged 6–12 years and 1200 mg/day in patients
aged 13 and above. Baseline studies prior to initiating treatment with
carbamazepine should include: general medical history and physical
examination; complete blood count with differential; liver function
tests; and a pregnancy test for sexually active females.

Possible common side-effects of carbamazepine in children and adolescents include sedation, ataxia, dizziness, blurred vision, nausea, and
vomiting. Because of its stimulation of the hepatic P-450 system, carbamazepine has many clinically significant drug interactions in children
and adolescents. Medications that will increase carbamazepine levels
include: erythromycin, cimetidine, fluoxetine, verapamil and valproate.
Carbamazepine may decrease the levels of the following medications:
phenobarbital, primidone, phenytoin, tricyclics, birth control pills and

lamotrigine. Carbamazepine is contraindicated in patients with a previous history of bone-marrow suppression or drug-induced hematological reactions. Rare cases of aplastic anemia and agranulocytosis have occurred with carbamazepine use and because of this, it is recommended that white blood cell counts be monitored carefully during the start of treatment with carbamazepine and that patients should be told to contact their physician if there are any signs of hematological problems including easy bruising, fever, sore throat or mouth ulcers.

Oxcarbazepine has a better safety profile than carbamazepine but potential side-effects also include somnolence, headache, dizziness, ataxia and diplopia. Like carbamazepine, hyponatremia may occur with oxcarbazepine treatment. However, oxcarbazepine is less likely to be associated with a rash than carbamazepine. Oxcarbazepine may diminish the efficacy of oral contraceptive medications. Table 7.2 lists the pediatric dosages, target serum levels, side-effects and cautions of lithium, valproate, carbamazepine, oxcarbazepine, and the miscellaneous mood stabilizers discussed below.

## Miscellaneous mood stabilizers

Recently, several new anti-seizure agents have been introduced which may also have mood-stabilizing properties. These agents include gabapentin (Neurontin®), lamotrigine (Lamictal®) and topiramate (Topamax®). Gabapentin was approved in the USA in 1994 for the treatment of adults who have partial seizures, either alone or with secondarily generalized seizures. Gabapentin is structurally similar to the inhibitory neurotransmitter gamma-aminobutyric acid (GABA) but its mechanism of action in humans is largely unknown. Several recent controlled studies of gabapentin as adjunctive therapy and as monotherapy found that it was no more effective than placebo for the treatment of adults with mania (Keck et al 2000; McElroy and Keck 2000). However, gabapentin may be useful in the treatment of the comorbid anxiety disorders frequently seen in BPD (Blanco et al 2002). One caution is that one of gabapentin's potential adverse effects in children is behavioral

Table 7.2 Mood stabilizers often used for bipolar children and adolescents

| Generic name | US trade name | How supplied (mg) | Starting dose | Target dose | Therapeutic serum level | Cautions |
|---|---|---|---|---|---|---|
| Carbamazepine | Tegretol | 100, 200 | Outpatients: | Based on | 4–11 mg/l | Watch for P-450-related |
| Carbamazepine XR | Tegretol XR | 100, 200, 400 | 7 mg/kg/day 2–3 daily doses | response and serum levels | | drug interactions, avoid pregnancy |
| Gabapentin | Neurontin | 100, 300, 400 | 100 mg BID or TID | Based on response | NA | Watch for behavioral disinhibition |
| Lamotrigine | Lamictal | 25, 100, 200 | 12.5 mg QD | Increase very slowly or bi-weekly based on response | NA | Monitor carefully for rashes, serum sickness |
| Li⁺carbonate | Lithobid | 300 (& 150 generic) | Outpatients: | 30 mg/kg/day | 0.8–1.2 mEq/l | Monitor for hypothyroidism |
| Li⁺carbonate | Eskalith | 300 or 450 CR | 25 mg/kg/day | 2–3 daily doses | | Avoid in pregnancy |
| Li⁺citrate | Cibaltih-S | Li-citrate 5 cc = 300 mg | 2–3 daily doses | | | |
| Oxcarbazepine | Trileptal | 150, 300, 600 | 150 mg BID | 20–29 kg 900 mg/day 30–39 kg 1200 mg/day >39 kg 1800 mg/day | NA | Monitor for hyponatremia |
| Topiramate | Topamax | 25, 100 | 25 mg QD | 100–400 mg/day | NA | Monitor for weight loss, memory problems, kidney stones |
| Valproic acid Divalproex sodium | Depakene Depakote | 125, 250, 500 | Outpatients: 15 mg/kg/day 2–3 daily doses | 20 mg/kg/day 2–3 daily doses | 85–110 mg/l | Monitor liver functions and for pancreatitis Avoid in pregnancy |

NA = not applicable

disinhibition. There are several case reports of this occurring in pediatric patients treated with gabapentin for seizure disorders (Lee et al 1996).

Lamotrigine is another anticonvulsant agent that was recently approved in the USA as an adjunctive agent in the treatment of adults who have partial seizures. Like gabapentin, there have also been several reports of lamotrigine's effectiveness in treating adults with BPD (Calabrese et al 1999; 2000). However, due the high incidence (1/100) of serious skin rashes, some of which progress to Stevens–Johnson syndrome, in 1998 the FDA issued a 'black-box' warning against using lamotrigine in patients below the age of 16 years. (Dooley et al 1996; Chaffin and Davis 1997; Fogh and Mai 1997) Since that time, the manufacturer has recommended a much more conservative titration schedule that has reduced the incidence of serious reactions to 1 in 2500 children. However, due to lamotrigine's lack of current FDA approval for psychiatric indications and the FDA's warning concerning it's use in pediatric populations, it must be used very carefully, if at all, in children and adolescents with BPD.

Topiramate is another anticonvulsant agent that may be effective in BPD. It has several mechanisms of action, including antagonism of the kainate/AMPA subtype of glutamate receptor, blockade of voltage-gated sodium channels, and carbonic anhydrase inhibition. Preliminary data from open studies suggest that topiramate may have mood-stabilizing properties in bipolar adults (McElroy et al 2000). There are no published, controlled trials of topiramate for the treatment of BPD in adults, children, or adolescents. Side-effects of topiramate include parasthesias, impaired concentration, and fatigue. In contrast to other mood stabilizers, topiramate is associated with anorexia and weight loss and this effect can sometimes be taken advantage of in patients who have a tendency to gain weight with other mood stabilizers. Word-finding and other cognitive difficulties have been reported in adult patients treated with topiramate, and this has also been reported to occur in children (Davanzo et al 2001).

## Summary

The mood stabilizers utilized in adults many times are effective in treating children and adolescents with pediatric bipolar disorders. However, controlled trials are necessary to determine their efficacy, alone and in combination, for children with the illness.

## Further reading

Alessi N, Naylor MW, Ghaziuddin M, Zubieta JK (1994) Update on lithium carbonate therapy in children and adolescents. *J Am Acad Child Adolesc Psychiatry* **33**: 291–304.

Bendz H., Aurell M, Balldin J et al (1994) Kidney damage in long-term lithium patients: a cross-sectional study of patients with 15 years or more on lithium. *Nephrol Dial Transplant* **9**: 1250–4.

Bendz H, Sjodin I, Aurell M (1996a) Renal function on and off lithium in patients treated with lithium for 15 years or more. A controlled, prospective lithium-withdrawal study. *Nephrol Dial Transplant* **11**: 457–60.

Bendz H, Sjodin I, Toss G, Berglund K. (1996b) Hyperparathyroidism and long-term lithium therapy–a cross-sectional study and the effect of lithium withdrawal. *J Int Med* **240**: 357–65.

Blanco C, Antia SX, Liebowitz MR (2002) Pharmacotherapy of social anxiety disorder. *Bio Psychiatry* **51**: 109–20.

Bowden CL (1996) Dosing strategies and time course of response to antimanic drugs. *J Clin Psychiatry* **57**: 4–9; discussion 10–2.

Cade JFJ (1949) Lithium salts in the treatment of psychotic excitement. *Med J Aust* **36**: 349–52.

Calabrese J, Bowden C, Sachs G et al (1999) A double-blind placebo-controlled study of lamotrigine monotherapy in outpatients with bipolar I depression. Lamictal 602 Study Group. *J Clin Psychiatry* **60**: 79–88.

Calabrese JR, Suppes T, Bowden, CL et al (2000) A double-blind, placebo-controlled, prophylaxis study of lamotrigine in rapid-cycling bipolar disorder. Lamictal 614 Study Group. *J Clin Psychiatry,* **61**, 841–50 [MEDLINE record in process].

Chaffin JJ, Davis SM (1997) Suspected lamotrigine-induced toxic epidermal necrolysis. *Ann Pharmacother* **31**: 720–3.

Chuang DM, Chen RW, Chalecha-Franaszek E et al (2002) Neuroprotective effects of lithium in cultured cells and animal models of disease. *Bipolar Disord* **4**: 129–36.

Ciraulo DA, Shader R J, Greenblatt DJ, Creelman W L (Eds) (1995) *Drug interactions in psychiatry,* Baltimore MD: Williams & Wilkins.

Cloyd JC, Fischer JH, Kriel RL, Kraus DM (1993) Valproic acid pharmacokinetics in children. IV. Effects of age and antiepileptic drugs on protein binding and intrinsic clearance. *Clin Pharmacol Ther* **53**: 22–9.

Cohen LS, Friedman JM, Jefferson JW et al (1994) A reevaluation of risk of in utero exposure to lithium. *JAMA* **271**: 146–50.

Cueva JE, Overall JE, Small AM et al (1996) Carbamazepine in aggressive children with conduct disorder: a double-blind and placebo-controlled study. *J Am Acad Child Adolesc Psychiatry* **35**: 480–90.

Davanzo P, Cantwell E, Kleiner J et al (2001) Cognitive changes during topiramate therapy. *J Am Acad Child Adolesc Psychiatry* **40**: 262–3.

DelBello M, Schweirs M, Rosenberg H et al (2002) Quetiapine as adjunctive treatment for adolescent mania associated with bipolar disorder. *J Am Acad Child Adolosc Psychiatry* (in press).

DelBello M, Schwiers M, Rosenberg H, Strakowski S (2001) Quetiapine as an adjunctive treatment for adolescent mania associated with bipolar disorder. *Archives of General Psychiatry (submitted)*.

Delong GR, Nieman MA (1983) Lithium-induced behavior changes in children with symptoms suggesting manic-depressive illness. *Psychopharm Bull* **19**: 258–65.

Deltito JA, Levitan J, Damore J et al (1998) Naturalistic experience with the use of divalproex sodium on an in-patient unit for adolescent psychiatric patients. *Acta Psychiatr Scand* **97**: 236–40.

Dooley J, Camfield P, Gordon K et al (1996) Lamotrigine-induced rash in children. *Neurology* **46**: 240–2.

Emrich HM, Dose M, von Zerssen D (1985) The use of sodium valproate, carbamazepine and oxcarbazepine in patients with affective disorders. *J Affect Disorders* **8**: 243–50.

Evans RW, Clay TH, Gualtieri CT (1987) Carbemazapine in pediatric psychiatry. *J Am Acad Child Adolesc Psychiatry* **26**: 2–8.

Fogh K, Mai J (1997) Toxic epidermal necrolysis after treatment with lamotrigine (Lamictal *Seizure* **6**: 63–5.

Geller B, Cooper TB, Sun K et al (1998) Double-blind and placebo-controlled study of lithium for adolescenet bipolar disorders with secondary substance dependency. *J Am Acad Child Adolesc Psychiatry* **37**: 171–78.

Gram LF, Rafaelsen OJ (1972) Lithium treatment of psychotic children and adolescents. A controlled clinical trial. *Acta Psychiatrica Scandinavica* **48**: 253–60.

Hirschfeld RMA (1994) *Am J Psychiatry* **151**: 1–36.

Isojarvi JI, Laatikainen TJ, Knip M et al (1996) Obesity and endocrine disorders in women taking valproate for epilepsy. *Ann Neurology* **39**: 579–84.

Isojarvi JI, Laatikainen TJ, Pakarinen AJ et al (1993) Polycystic ovaries and hyperandrogenism in women taking valproate for epilepsy. *N Engl J Med* **329**: 1383–8.

Janicak PG, Davis JM, Preskorn SH, Ayd FJ (1993) *Principles and Practice of Psychopharmacotherapy*. Baltimore, MD: Williams & Wilkins.

Kafantaris V (1995) Treatment of bipolar disorder in children and adolescents. *J Am Acad Child Adolesc Psychiatry* **34**: 732–41.

Kafantaris V, Campbell M, Padron-Gayol MV et al (1992) Carbamazepine in hospitalized aggressive conduct disorder children: an open pilot study. *Psychopharmacol Bull* **28**: 193–9.

Kastner F, Friedman DL (1992) Verapamil and valproic acid treatment of prolonged mania. *J Am Acad Child Adolesc Psychiatry* **31**: 271–75.

Kastner F, Friedman DL, Plummer AT et al (1990) Valproic acid for the treatment of children with mental retardation and mood symptomatology. *Pediatrics* **86:** 467–72.

Keck PE Jr, McElroy SL, Nemeroff CB (1992) Anticonvulsants in the treatment of bipolar disorder. *J Neuropsychiatry Clin Neurosci* **4:** 395–405.

Keck PJ, Mendlwicz J, Calabrese J et al (2000) *J Affect Disord* **59** Suppl 1: S31–S37.

Kowatch RA, Suppes T, Carmody TJ et al (2000) Effect size of lithium, divalproex sodium, and carbamazepine in children and adolescents with bipolar disorder. *J Am Acad Child Adolesc Psychiatry* **39:** 713–20.

Lee DO, Steingard RJ, Cesena M et al (1996) Behavioral side effects of gabapentin in children. *Epilepsia* **37:** 87–90.

Lena B (1979) Lithium in child and adolescent psychiatry. *Arch Gen Psychiatry* **36:** 854–5.

Loscher W (1993) Effects of the antiepileptic drug valproate on metabolism and function of inhibitory and excitatory amino acids in the brain. *Neurochem Res* **18:** 485–502.

Luef G, Abraham I, Trinka E et al (2001) Weight change associated with valproate and lamotrigine monotherapy in patients with epilepsy. *Neurology* **57:** 565–6.

Manji HK, Chen G, Hsiao JK et al (1996) Regulation of signal transduction pathways by mood-stabilizing agents: implications for the delayed onset of therapeutic efficacy. *J Clin Psychiatry* **57:** 34–46; discussion 47–8.

McClellan J, Werry JS (1997) Practice parameters for the assessment and treatment of children and adolescents with bipolar disorder. *J Am Acad Child Adolesc Psychiatry* **36 (Suppl)** : 157S–176S.

McElroy SL, Keck PE.Jr (2000) Pharmacologic agents for the treatment of acute bipolar mania. *Biol Psychiatry* **48:** 539–57.

McElroy SL, Suppes T, Keck PE et al (2000) Open-label adjunctive topiramate in the treatment of bipolar disorders. *Biol Psychiatry* **47:** 1025–33.

McKnew DH, Cytryn L, Buchsbaum MS et al (1981) Lithium in children of lithium-responding parents. *Psychiatry Res* **4:** 171–80.

Nau H, Hauck RS, Ehlers K (1991) Valproic acid-induced neural tube defects in mouse and human: aspects of chirality, alternative drug development, pharmacokinetics and possible mechanisms. *Pharmacol Toxicol* **69:** 310–21.

Papatheodorou G, Kutcher SP (1993) Divalproex sodium treatment in late adolescent and young adult acute mania. *Psychopharmacol Bull* **29:** 213–9.

Papatheodorou G, Kutcher SP, Katic M, Szalai JP (1995) The efficacy and safety of divalproex sodium in the treatment of acute mania in adolescents and young adults: an open clinical trial. *J Clin Psychopharmacol* **15:** 110–6.

Post RM, Ketter TA, Denicoff K et al (1996) The place of anticonvulsant therapy in bipolar illness. *Psychopharmacology (Berl)* **128:** 115–29.

Puente RM (1975) In *Epileptic seizures – behaviour – pain* (W Birkmayer, ed.) Baltimore, MD: University Park Press, pp. 243–52.

Rasgon NL, Altshuler LL, Gudeman D (2000) Medication status and polycystic ovary syndrome in women with bipolar disorder: a preliminary report. *J Clin Psychiatry* **61:** 173–8.

Reischer H, Pfeffer CR (1996) Lithium pharmacokinetics. *J Am Acad Child Adolesc Psychiatry* **35:** 130–1.

Rimmer EM, Richens A (1985) An update on sodium valproate. *Pharmacotherapy* **5:** 171–84.

Vitiello B, Behar D, Malone R et al (1988) Pharmacokinetics of lithium carbonate in children. *J Clin Psychopharmacol* **8**: 355–9.

Wagner KD, Weller E, Biederman J et al (2001) In *47th Annual Meeting of the American Academy of Child and Adolescent Psychiatry*, New York, p. 116.

Weller EB, Weller RA, Fristad MA (1986) Lithium dosage guide for prepubertal children: a preliminary report. *J Am Acad Child Psychiatry* **25**: 92–5.

West K., McElroy SL (1995) Oral loading doses in the valproate treatment of adolescents with mixed bipolar disorder. *J Child Adolesc Psychopharmacology* **5**: 225–31.

West SA, Keck PEJ, McElroy SL et al (1994) Open trial of valproate in the treatment of adolescent mania. *J Child Adolesc Psychopharmacol* **4**: 263–67.

# chapter 8

# Atypical antipsychotics in the treatment of pediatric bipolar disorders

Evidence for the use of atypical antipsychotics in BPD

The atypical antipsychotics are powerful psychotropic agents that have recently been found to be efficacious in the treatment of adults with schizophrenia and acute mania (Glick et al 2001; Kapur and Remington 2001). The atypical antipsychotics differ from typical antipsychotics in their 'limbic–specific' dopamine type 2 (D2)-receptor binding and high ratio of serotonin type 2 (5-HT2)-receptor binding to D2 binding (Gupta and Masand 1997). The mechanism of action of these drugs involves antagonism of several receptors in the brain: serotonin $5HT_{1A}$ and $5HT_2$, dopamine D1 and D2, histamine H1, and adrenergic $alpha_1$ and $alpha_2$ . An overview of the differential receptor binding of several of these agents is illustrated in Figure 8.1.

The atypical antipsychotics not only have antipsychotic activity but may also possess thymoleptic properties with favorable effects on depressive and manic symptoms of patients with bipolar disorders (Keck 2001). To date, there have been three large controlled studies of olanzapine (Berk et al 1999; Tohen et al 1999; 2000), two trials of risperidone (Segal et al 1998; Sachs 1999), and one trial of ziprasidone in the

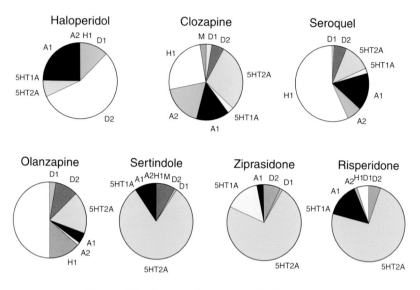

**Figure 8.1** *Comparative receptor binding profiles*

treatment of BPD adults. All of these studies found these atypical agents to be efficacious for the treatment of mania in adults. The results of these adult mania studies with atypical antipsychotics studies are summarized in Table 8.1.

Ziprasidone (Geodon) is another recently-developed atypical antipsychotic that has demonstrated efficacy in reducing positive and negative symptoms, and symptoms of depression in schizophrenia during both short- and long-term clinical trials in adults (Keck et al 2001). Ziprasidone like other atypical antipsychotics has combined dopamine and serotonin receptor antagonist activity and its most potent action is at the 5-HT2A site. Ziprasidone does not cause any known hematological problems or seizures, is less sedating than other antipsychotics, and does not cause the weight gain seen with other atypical antipsychotic agents (Weiden 2001). Keck and colleagues recently reviewed the data from two separate multi-center trials of schizophrenic adults that also included patients with schizoaffective disorder (Keck et al 2001). In these two

Table 8.1  Studies of atypical antipsychotics in adult bipolar mania

| Study (see Further Reading section) | Design | n | Mean age (years) | Trial duration (days) | Primary efficacy measure | Response rate by intent-to-treat sample | Control event rate (CER) |
|---|---|---|---|---|---|---|---|
| Segal et al 1998 | Random, Parallel-Group: Risperidone Haloperidol Lithium | 45 | 33.6 | 28 | BPRS Y-MRS CGIS GAF SAS | Not reported  All groups significant. improved on Y-MRS (p<.001) | NA |
| Tohen et al 1999 | Random, PBO, Parallel-Group: Olanz PBO | 139 | 39.5 | 21 | >50% Change from baseline in Y-MRS | Olanz. 48% | PBO 23% |
| Tohen et al 2000 | Random, PBO, Parallel-Group: Olanz PBO | 115 | 39 | 28 | >50% Change from baseline in Y-MRS | Olanz. 65% | PBO 43% |
| Keck et al 2000 | Random, PBO, Parallel-Group: Zipras. PBO | 195 | NA | 21 | >50% Change from baseline in Y-MRS | Zipras. 50% | PBO 36% |

controlled trials there were 115 adult inpatients with schizoaffective disorder that were treated with ziprasidone. These subjects were diagnosed with DSM-IIIR schizoaffective disorder, bipolar or depressive type and their mean age was 38 years. The authors concluded that both ziprasidone, 120 mg/day, and 160 mg/day, were significantly more effective than placebo on all the primary efficacy measures. The most common side-effects reported were somnolence and headaches.

Recently Keck and colleagues reported the results of a controlled trial of ziprasidone in adult inpatients with BPD (Keck et al 2000). In this 3-week, controlled trial, 195 inpatients, were randomized to ziprasidone, 80–160 mg/day, or placebo. They reported that 'Robust improvements in the MRS score were observed with ziprasidone compared to placebo at all timepoints after baseline.' Ziprasidone appears to be as effective as the other atypical antipsychotic agents in the treatment of BPD in adults.

Another atypical is expected to be FDA approved for adults in 2003. Aripiperazole acts differently to other drugs in this class as it is a partial agonist at D2, D3 and 5HT1A receptors, rather than a full antagonist. Data from trials in adult patients with schizophrenia indicate a good side-effects profile with excellent tolerability and no weight gain.

## Atypical antipsychotics: child and adolescent BPD studies

There have been no placebo-controlled studies of atypical antipsychotics in pediatric BPD patients, but there have been several recent case series and open-label reports suggesting that atypical agents such as clozapine (Kowatch et al 1995), risperidone (Frazier et al 1999) and olanzapine (Soutullo et al 1999; Chang and Ketter 2000; Khouzam and Gabalawi 2000) are effective in the treatment of pediatric BPD. In a retrospective case series of severely ill children and adolescents (5/10 of whom were diagnosed with bipolar disorder), Kowatch et al reported that these subject's CGI severity ratings significantly improved from baseline to endpoint, suggesting that clozapine may be effective for treatment resistant pediatric BPD. Besides the risk of agranulocytosis, clozapine causes large weight gains and significant sedation in the majority of pediatric BPD patients. In a retrospective chart review of outpatients ($n = 28$), Frazier and colleagues investigated the effectiveness and tolerability of adjunctive risperidone for the treatment of pediatric mania (Frazier et al 1999). The authors used the Clinical Global Impression Scale (CGI) with separate assessments of mania, psychosis, aggression, and attention-deficit/hyperactivity disorder (ADHD). These children received a mean dose of $1.7 \pm 1.3$ mg over an average period of $6.1 \pm 8.5$ months. Using a CGI Improvement score of $\leq 2$ (very much/much improved) to define robust improvement, 82% showed improvement in both their manic and aggressive symptoms, 69% in psychotic symptoms, but only 8% in ADHD symptoms. Although this study is limited by its retrospective nature, these data suggest that risperidone may be effective for the treatment of pediatric as well as adult mania.

Several case series and reports have indicated that olanzapine, may be useful for the treatment of mania associated with pediatric BPD (Soutullo et al 1999; Chang and Ketter 2000; Khouzam and Gabakawi 2000). However, most of these reports are retrospective and the total number of subjects is small ($n = 11$). In a more recent study, Frazier and colleagues reported the effectiveness and tolerability of olanzapine for the treatment of acute mania in children and adolescents (Frazier et al 2001). The study was an 8-week open label prospective study of olanzapine monotherapy (dose range 2.5–20 mg/day) for the treatment of 23 bipolar children and adolescents. Using a predefined criterion for improvement of >30% decline in Y-MRS and a CGI-S mania score of <3 at endpoint, the overall response rate was 61%. Overall, olanzapine was fairly well tolerated, however, body weight increased significantly during the 8-week study.

Table 8.2 summarizes the two recent trials of atypical antipsychotics in children and adolescents with BPD. Both of these studies found significant effects for the atypical agent used. DelBello et al (2001) (discussed in Chapter 7) found that the combination of a mood stabilizer and an atypical antipsychotic agent produced a better response rate than only a mood stabilizer for the treatment of mania in children and adolescents with BPD.

Table 8.2 Atypical studies in BPD children and adolescents

| Study (see Further Reading section) | Design | n | Mean age (years) | Trial duration (days) | Primary efficacy measure | Response rate by intent-to-treat sample | Control event rate (CER) |
|---|---|---|---|---|---|---|---|
| Frazier et al 2001 | Open-label prospective monotherapy | 23 | 10.3 | 56 | > 30% change from baseline in Y-MRS and CGI severity score ≤3 | 61% | NA |
| DelBello et al 2002 | Random, parallel group: DVP + PBO or DVP + Quetiapine | 30 | 14 | 42 | > 50% change from baseline in Y-MRS | Quetiapine + DVP 87% | DVP + PBO 53% |

# Clinical use of atypical antipsychotics

It has recently become apparent that ziprasidone and several other antipsychotic agents can prolong the QT interval which could potentially cause malignant ventricular arrhythmias like Torsades de pointes (Welch and Chue 2000). The QT interval reflects the time of electrical impulses from the start of ventricular depolarization to repolarization, the stage that prepares the ventricles for the next beat. The repolarization/depolarization process must accelerate as the heart rate increases, and the corrected QT (QTc) interval adjusts for this difference. In recently considering a new drug application for the antipsychotic ziprasidone, the US Food and Drug Administration (FDA) required a study of the propensity of the drug to prolong QTc interval relative to other antipsychotics. This study protocol involved measuring changes in QTc interval from baseline to that occurring at the peak serum level of dosages required for controlling symptoms of schizophrenia. These changes were then ascertained in both the absence and presence of interacting medications that inhibited metabolism of the respective antipsychotics. The study revealed that ziprasidone causes a 9–14 ms greater mean prolongation in QTc than four of the comparator drugs (risperidone, olanzapine, quetiapine or haloperidol); but approximately 14 ms less than the other comparator drug (thioridazine) (Pfizer 2000). EKG monitoring at baseline and with each major dose increase of an atypical antipsychotic may be indicated when these agents are used to treat children and adolescents with BPD.

Table 8.3 lists the pediatric dosages, target serum levels, side-effects and cautions of the atypical antipsychotic agents discussed below.

## Risperidone

Risperidone (Risperdal) is an atypical antipsychotic agent that was introduced in the USA in 1994. Risperidone is indicated in the USA for the management of psychotic conditions and its antipsychotic activity appears to be mediated through a combination of dopamine type 2 (D2) and serotonin type 2 (5HT2) antagonism.

Risperidone is extensively metabolized in the liver by cytochrome

Table 8.3 Atypical antipsychotic agents in children and adolescents with BPD

| Generic name | Trade name | How supplied (mg) | Starting dose | Target dose (mg/Day) | Cautions |
|---|---|---|---|---|---|
| Clozapine | Clozaril | 25, 100 | 25 BID | 200–400 | Monitor WBC weekly Seizures possible at higher doses |
| Olanzapine | Zyprexa Zydis | 2.5, 5, 7.5, 10 5 | 2.5 BID | 10–20 | Monitor weight |
| Quetiapine | Seroquel | 25, 100, 200 | 25 BID | 200–600 | Periodic eye examination is recommended |
| Risperidone | Risperdal | 0.25, 0.5, 1,2, 3, 4 | 0.25 BID | 1–2 | Monitor for EPS and galactorrhea |
| Ziprasidone | Geodon | 20, 40, 60, 80 | 20 BID | 80–120 | Check baseline EKG |

P-450IID6 to a major active metabolite, 9-hydroxyrisperidone, which is equivalent to risperidone with respect to receptor binding activity.

Risperidone is very potent at low doses, 0.25–2.0 mg/day, and can cause extrapyramidal symptoms at higher doses, e.g. >2 mg/day. It can also cause tardive dyskinesia (Haberfellner 1997), neuroleptic malignant syndrome, and there are several case reports of the induction of mania at higher doses (Koek and Kessler 1996; Schnierow and Graeber 1996; Barkin et al 1997). Possible side effects of risperidone include sedation, weight gain, drooling, night terrors and galactorrhea.

Risperdal tablets are available in 0.25 mg (dark yellow), 0.5 mg (red–brown), 1 mg (white), 2 mg (orange), 3 mg (yellow), and 4 mg (green) strengths. A typical starting dose of risperidone in children or adolescents with BPD would be 0.25 mg twice daily with dosage increases every 3–5 days as based on a patient's symptomatic response. A target dose of risperidone in manic children is in the range of 1–2 mg/day.

## Olanzapine

Olanzapine (Zyprexa/Zydis) was introduced to the USA in 1996 and is indicated by the FDA for the long-term therapy and maintenance of treatment response of schizophrenia and the short-term treatment of acute manic episodes associated with bipolar I disorder. Like most atypical antipsychotics, it is thought that olanzapine's antipsychotic activity is mediated through a combination of dopamine and serotonin type 2 (5HT2) antagonism. Olanzapine's antagonism of muscarinic M1-5 receptors may explain its anticholinergic effects and its antagonism of histamine H1 receptors may explain the somnolence and weight gain observed with it. Olanzapine is well absorbed and reaches peak concentrations in approximately 6 hours following an oral dose. Olanzapine displays linear kinetics over the clinical dosing range and its half-life in adults ranges from 21 to 54 hours. Direct glucuronidation and cytochrome P-450 (CYP)-mediated oxidation are the primary metabolic pathways for olanzapine.

Possible side-effects of olanzapine include sedation, weight gain, runny nose, dizziness and headache. Olanzapine is available as white, film-coated tablets imprinted in blue ink with LILLY and the tablet number. Four tablet strengths of olanzapine are available: 2.5 mg, 5 mg, 7.5 mg, and 10 mg. Olanzapine is also available as an orally disintegrating tablets (Zydis®) that dissolves in the mouth on contact with saliva. Zydis is available in 5 mg and 10 mg tablets. A typical starting dose of olanzapine for a manic child is 2.5 mg twice daily with dosage increases every 3–5 days based on a patient's symptomatic response. A target dose of olanzapine is in the range of 10–20 mg/day. Zydis is very effective as a 'PRN' medication in pediatric patients who become very agitated or psychotic when manic.

## Quetiapine

Quetiapine (Seroquel) was approved by the FDA in 1997 for the treatment of acute and chronic psychoses, including schizophrenia. Like the other atypical antipsychotics, quetiapine has a broad receptor binding profile, with an affinity for 5-HT2 receptors and D2 receptors. Quetiapine is well absorbed and extensively metabolized following oral administration. The bioavailability of quetiapine is not significantly affected by administration with food. The elimination half-life of quetiapine in adults is approximately 7 hours. Quetiapine and several of its metabolites are weak inhibitors of human cytochrome P-450 1A2, 2C9, 2C19, 2D6 and 3A4 activities, but only at concentrations at least 10- to 50-fold higher than those observed at the usual effective dose range of 300–450 mg/day in humans. Based on these in vitro results, it is unlikely that coadministration of quetiapine with other drugs will result in clinically significant drug inhibition of cytochrome P-450-mediated metabolism of the other drug.

Possible side-effects of quetiapine include sedation, hypotension, constipation, dry mouth and dizziness. In our experience, quetiapine may not cause as much weight gain as olanzapine and risperidone. Quetiapine can cause cataracts in animals but this has not been observed in human subjects. Quetiapine is available in tablet strengths of 25 mg (peach), 100 mg (yellow), 200 mg (white) and 300 mg (white oval) tablets.

A typical starting dose of quetiapine for a manic child is 25 mg twice daily with dosage increases every 3–5 days based on a patient's symptomatic response. A target dose of quetiapine in manic children is in the range of 200–600 mg/day.

## Ziprasidone

Ziprasidone (Geodon) was approved by the FDA in 2001 for treatment of schizophrenia and schizoaffective disorder. Ziprasidone produces its effect as an antagonist at the dopamine (D2) and serotonin (5HT2A, 5HT1D) receptor subtypes. It also inhibits re-uptake of both serotonin and norepinephrine. In addition, it demonstrates activity at histamine (H1) receptors contributing to sedation and activity at alpha-receptors resulting in orthostatic hypotension.

Ziprasidone's activity is primarily due to the parent drug and it is well absorbed after oral administration, reaching peak plasma concentrations in 6–8 hours. Elimination of ziprasidone is mainly via hepatic metabolism with a mean terminal half-life of about 7 hours in adults. Steady-state concentrations are achieved within 1–3 days of dosing. Ziprasidone is unlikely to interfere with the metabolism of drugs metabolized by cytochrome P-450 enzymes.

As mentioned above, ziprasidone may cause QTc prolongation and if there is a family history of sudden cardiac death, get an EKG before starting ziprasidone, and obtain a repeat EKG at each significant dose increase. Certain conditions may predispose a patient at risk to these cardiac effects including hypokalemia, hypomagnesemia, bradycardia, or genetic predisposition to prolonged QTc intervals. Ziprasidone is contraindicated in patients with a known history of QT prolongation (including congenital long QT syndrome). In addition, medications known to prolong the QTc interval include antiarrthymics, tricyclic antidepressants, antipsychotics, macrolide antibiotics, and certain fluoroquinolones; their concurrent use with ziprasidone should be avoided.

Ziprasidone is available as capsules in 20 mg (blue/white), 40 mg (blue/blue), 60 mg (white/white), and 80 mg (blue/white) dosages. A typical starting dose of ziprasidone for a manic child is 20 mg twice daily with dosage increases every 3–5 days based on a patient's symptomatic response. A target dose of ziprasidone for manic children is in the range of 80–120 mg/day.

# Summary

The atypical antipsychotics are potent agents that have antipsychotic and antimanic properties. Their use in bipolar children and adolescents, however, must be tempered by their serious side-effects, which often include weight gain and sedation, and a lack of studies of their anti-depressant and long term mood-stabilizing effects in children.

# Further reading

Barkin JS, Pais VM Jr, Gaffney MF (1997) Induction of mania by risperidone resistant to mood stabilizers. *J Clin Psychopharmacol* **17**: 57–8.

Berk M, Ichim L, Brook S (1999) Olanzapine compared to lithium in mania: a double-blind randomized controlled trial. *Int Clin Pyschopharmacol* **14**: 339–43.

Chang K, Ketter T (2000) Mood stabilizer augmentation with olanzapine in acutely manic children. *J Child Adolesc Psychopharmacol* **10**: 45–9.

DelBello M, Schwiers M, Rosenberg H, Strakowski S (2001) Risperidone treatment for juvenile bipolar disorder: a retrospective chart review. *Arch Gen Psychiatry (submitted)*.

Frazier J, Meyer M, Biederman J (1999) *J Am Soc Child Adolesc Psychiatry* **38**: 960–5.

Frazier JA, Biederman J, Jacobs TG et al (2001) A prospective open-label treatment trial of olanzapine monotherapy in children and adolescents with bipolar disorder. *J of Child Adolesc Psychopharm* **11**: 239–50.

Glick I, Murray S, Vasudevan P et al (2001) Treatment with atypical antipsychotics: new indications and new populations. *J Psychiatric Res* **35**: 187–91.

Gupta S, Masand P (1997) Olanzapine: Review of its pharmacology and indication in clinical practice. *Primary Psychiatry* 73–82.

Haberfellner EM (1997) Tardive dyskinesia during treatment with risperidone. *Pharmacopsychiatry* **30**: 271.

Kapur S, Remington G (2001) Atypical antipsychotics: new directions and new challenges in the treatment of schizophrenia. *Ann Rev med* **52**: 503–17.

Keck P, Ice K, Ziprasidone MSG (2000) A 3-week, double-blind, randomized trial of ziprasidone in the acute treatment of mania. *40th Annual NCDEU*. Boca Raton, FL: NIMH.

Keck PE (2001) Atypical antipsychotics as mood stabilizers. by Arline Kaplan

Keck PJ, McElroy S, Arnold L (2001a) Ziprasidone: a new atypical antipsychotic. *Expert Opin Pharmacother* **2**: 1033–42.

Keck PJ, Reeves K, Harrigan E (2001b) Ziprasidone in the short-term treatment of patients with schizoaffective disorder: results from two double-blind, placebo-controlled, multicenter studies. *J Clin Psychopharmacology* **21**: 27–35.

Khouzam H, E-Gabalawi F (2000) Treatment of bipolar I disorder in an adolescent with olanzapine. *J Child Adolesc Psychoharmacology* **10**: 147–51.

Koek RJ, Kessler CC (1996) Probable induction of mania by risperidone. *J Clin Psychiatry* **57**: 174–5.

Kowatch RA, Suppes T, Gilfillan SK et al (1995) Treatment of children and adolescents with bipolar disorder and schizophrenia. *J of Child Adolesc Psychopharm* **5**: 241–53.

Pfizer I. (2000) Pfizer FDA brieifing document for Zeldox capsules (ziprasidone). New York, p. 116.

Sachs GS (1999) *38th Annual meeting of the American College of Neuropharmacology.* Acapulco, Mexico.

Schnierow BJ, Graeber DA (1996) Manic symptoms associated with initiation of risperidone. *Am J Psychiatry* **153**: 1235–6.

Segal J, Berk M, Brook S (1998) Risperidone compared with both lithium and haloperidol in mania: a double-blind randomized controlled trial. *Clin Neuropharmacol* **21**: 176–80.

Soutullo C, Sorter M, Foster K et al (1999) Olanzapine in the treatment of adolescent acute mania: a report of seven cases. *J Affect Disord* **53**: 279–83.

Tohen M, Jacobs TG, Grundy SL et al (2000) Efficacy of olanzapine in acute bipolar mania: a double-blind, placebo-controlled study. The Olanzipine HGGW Study Group. *Arch Gen Psychiatry* **57**: 841–9.

Tohen M, Sanger T, McElroy S et al (1999) Olanzapine versus placebo in the treatment of acute mania. Olanzapine HGEH Study Group. *Am J Psychiatry* **156**: 702–9.

Weiden P (2001) A new atypical antipsychotic. *J Psychiatric Practice* 145–53.

Welch R, Chue P (2000) Antipsychotic agents and QT changes. *J Psychiatry Neurosci* **25**: 154–60.

# chapter 9

# Strategies and tactics in the treatment of children and adolescents with bipolar disorders

## Introduction

There have been several clinical practice guidelines recently published about the treatment of bipolar disorders (BPD) in adults (Suppes et al 1998; Bauer et al 1999; Goldberg 2000; Sachs et al 2000). These guidelines are useful as they offer a concise review of the bipolar treatment literature and summarize reasonable options for initiating and maintaining treatment in the various clinical scenarios common to bipolar disorders. Unfortunately, these guidelines were written for adults and the only set of guidelines specific to bipolar children and adolescents, American Academy of Child and Adolescent Psychiatry (AACAP) 1997 Practice Parameters For The Assessment And Treatment Of Children And Adolescents With Bipolar Disorder, are out-of-date and not comprehensive enough to be useful in most clinical situations (McClellan and Werry 1997). The general guidelines that we have developed for the treatment of children and adolescents are based on published adult guidelines, the emerging child and adolescent bipolar treatment literature, and our own clinical experience. These recommendations do not apply to all patients, and each should be modified and tailored to each individual patient.

The paradigm of 'strategies and tactics' was first used by John Rush to describe the principles of maintenance phase treatment for adults with major depressive disorder (Rush 1999). Rush defined strategies as 'what treatments to choose and in what order', and tactics as 'how to implement these strategies once chosen, in terms of dose and duration of treatment'. This is a very useful way of conceptualizing treatment that we have adapted for children and adolescents with bipolar disorders. For the purposes of this chapter we have defined the following terms:

- Strategies: An overall treatment plan that targets bipolar symptoms, e.g. decrease the number of mood swings per day using mood stabilizers.
- Tactics: What specific agents to use alone and in combination to achieve symptomatic remission and functional recovery with individual patients.

## Strategy1: Prior to treatment: perform a careful assessment

Specific Tactics: Confirm the diagnosis of bipolar disorder; the sub-type of BPD; assess comorbid disorders; the patient's family history; and medical and past treatment responses.

### Tactic 1: Confirm the diagnosis of bipolar disorder

The first tactic before initiating treatment is to verify that the patient you are considering for treatment has a bipolar illness. Many children and adolescents are labeled 'bipolar' without careful consideration of the diagnostic complexities and subtypes of this disorder, but more often the diagnosis is missed or overlooked. The symptoms of bipolarity in children and adolescents can be difficult to establish because of the effects of development upon symptom expression, the variability of symptom expression depending upon the context and phase of the illness, and other medications that the patient is currently taking. There are a number of medications and medical disorders that may mimic or exacerbate bipolar symptoms and it is important to assess these poten-

Table 9.1  Medical conditions and medications that may mimic
mania in children and adolescents

| Medical conditions | Medications |
| --- | --- |
| Alcohol related neurodevelopmental disorder | Antidepressants |
| Temporal lobe epilepsy | Psychomotor stimulants |
| Closed or open head injury | Steriods |
| Hyperthyroidism | |
| Multiple sclerosis | |
| Systemic lupus erythematosus | |
| Addison's disease | |
| Wilson's disease | |

tial confounds before initiating treatment. Potential rare medical disorders and common medications that should be considered in the differential diagnosis of a pediatric BPD are listed in Table 9.1. Prior to
treatment with any psychotropic agents, each patient should undergo a
medical history, medical review of systems, physical and appropriate
laboratory examinations.

### Tactic 2: Clarify the sub-type of BPD

It is important to clarify the episode presentation and bipolar subtype
and type of bipolar episode prior to beginning treatment, as this may
help determine which medications are used. The diagnostic classification system that DSM-IV uses for bipolar disorders is complex, involving
five types of episode (manic, hypomanic, mixed, depressed, unspecified),
four severity levels (mild, moderate, severe without psychosis, severe
with psychosis), and three course specifiers (with or without
interepisode recovery, seasonal pattern, rapid cycling). These DSM-IV
criteria were developed from data on adults with bipolar disorders and
none take into account developmental differences between bipolar
adults and bipolar children or adolescents. Pediatric bipolar patients
often present with a mixed or 'dysphoric' picture characterized by frequent short periods of intense mood liability and irritability rather than

classic euphoric mania. Clinicians who evaluate children with pediatric bipolar disorders often try to fit them into the DSM-IV 'rapid cycling' subtype and find that this subtype does not fit bipolar children very well as these children often do not have clear episodes of mania. Rather, researchers are reporting that bipolar children cycle far more frequently than four episodes per year with Geller and colleagues reporting continuous cycling from mania or hypomania to euthymia or depression in 81% of a well-defined samples of patients (Geller et al 1995). However, despite these differences in phenomenology, it is important to make a provisional subtype diagnosis (BP I, BP II, cyclothymia, or BP-NOS), before initiating treatment and then revising the diagnosis as additional prospective longitudinal observations and information become available.

### Tactic 3: Assess comorbid disorders

Children and adolescent with pediatric bipolar disorders often have comorbid disorders that complicate their treatment response. These comorbid disorders most often include attention-deficit hyperactivity disorder (ADHD), anxiety disorders, oppositional defiant disorder and conduct disorder (Kovacs and Pollock 1995; West et al 1995; Wozniak et al 1995). ADHD is the most common comorbid disorder among pediatric bipolar patients; leading research groups find comorbid rates as high as 98% (Wozniak et al 1995) and 97% (Geller et al 1998). Pediatric bipolar disorder with comorbid ADHD can be difficult to treat because of the fear of exacerbating the patient's mood disorder while treating their ADHD with stimulants. This is more likely to happen when mood stabilizers are not used first or concurrently. In 1992 Carlson and colleagues reported a 'synergistic rather than an antagonistic effect' of lithium and methylphenidate in seven hospitalized children with DSMIIIR BP-NOS disorder and disruptive behavior disorders (Carlson et al 1992). Biederman et al reported a series of 38 pediatric patients who were diagnosed with DSMIIIR mania and ADHD and treated first with mood stabilizers and then stimulants (Biederman et al 1999). They reported that those patients who first had their mania treated with mood stabilizers responded very well to the addition of a stimulant medication (Biederman et al 1999).

### Tactic 4: Assess the patient's family history

The patient's family history may offer clues to the diagnosis and perhaps treatment of BPD. Although few have studied whether a BPD parent's response to a specific agent predicts their child's response, it is often helpful to determine at what age the parent with BPD first became symptomatic, what their course has been and to what agents they did or did not respond. Parents that have been on various psychotropic medications for their own bipolar illnesses are often in a better position to monitor for treatment effects and side-effects. Moreover, Grof and colleagues have found that lithium response tends to run in families (Grof et al 1994).

### Tactic 5: Assess the patient's past treatment responses

It is important as part of the patient's psychiatric work-up to get a thorough history of what psychotropic medications the patient has been treated with in the past including the dosages, duration of treatment, tolerance, and effect on bipolar symptoms. It is surprising how often children and adolescents with prominent bipolar symptoms have been treated with every psychotropic agent except a mood stabilizer. Serotonin-selective re-uptake inhibitors (SSRIs) and stimulant medications in the absence of mood stabilizer may exacerbate bipolar symptoms, further clouding the picture of BPD. It is in many cases extremely helpful to taper medications that may exacerbate BPD over a short period of time – 1 or 2 weeks – and then revaluate the patient's symptoms. If the patient's BPD symptoms remain problematic, then aggressive treatment is warranted.

### Tactic 6: Identify BPD target symptoms

Pediatric BPD symptoms are different depending upon the patient, the phase of their illness and the bipolar subtype. It is important to differentiate the type of episode that the patient is currently experiencing and to identify the 'target symptoms' of this episode that are the most important to resolve with treatment. For many patients during a manic or mixed episode their cardinal symptoms include those such as dramatic rapid mood swings within a day, aggressive behavior and irritability. During a depressive episode symptoms may include decreased energy, social withdrawal, an increase in total sleep period and a change in appetite.

## Strategies and tactics for common pediatric BPD treatment scenarios

### The prepubertal, non-psychotic, 'complex-cycling' BPD patient

The prepubertal, non-psychotic, 'complex-cycling' patient is the most common and difficult type of pediatric bipolar patient to diagnose and treat. The parents or guardians of these patients typically report five–ten severe mood swings per day with almost constant mood cycling and no clear episodes, i.e. the complex cycling pattern of pediatric bipolars recently validated by Geller et al in several large, well-controlled, longitudinal samples (Geller et al 1995; Geller et al 2000). These patients have usually been treated with almost every medication except a mood stabilizer and have frequently not responded well to stimulants. They often have comorbid ADHD or anxiety disorders, and cycle continuously, without clear episodes of mania or depression.

The strategy with this type of BPD patient is to taper any medications that may be exacerbating their bipolar symptoms and initiate treatment with a mood stabilizer. This tapering can usually be done over a short period of time, 1 or 2 weeks. Most psychotropic medications can be safely tapered by halving the total daily dose every 3–5 days until the medication is discontinued and then the patient's BPD symptoms evaluated again.

In this scenario, it may be best to initiate treatment with valproate, titrate up according to therapeutic effects and tolerability, often to a serum level between 85 and 110 µg/ml, and then assess the patient's

---

Table 9.2  Medications that may increase mood cycling in children and adolescents

1. Tricyclic antidepressants
2. Serotonin-selective re-uptake inhibitors
3. Serotonin and norepinephrine re-uptake inhibitors
4. Corticosteroids
5. Aminophylline
6. Sympathomimetic amines (e.g. pseudoephedrine, etc.)

response after 3–6 weeks of treatment. Table 7.2 lists the mood stabilizing agents used most often to treat bipolar disorders and lists their pediatric dosages, target serum levels, side-effects and cautions.

If the patient shows only a partial response (slight to moderate improvement) to valproate after 3–6 weeks of treatment and is not psychotic, then adding lithium to valproate is in many cases helpful in eliciting a better response. Among adult bipolars, single mood stabilizers are usually not sufficient for achieving good for long-term treatment efficacy and often combination therapy with lithium, carbamazepine or divalproex sodium, and other agents is necessary (Post 1993; Prien and Rush 1996; Solomon et al 1996; Frye et al 2000). This is also true in many BPD children and adolescents who may require a combination of mood stabilizers to achieve behavioral control and euthymia. In the only well-controlled, prospective study of lithium carbonate in adolescents with bipolar disorder and comorbid substance abuse, Geller and colleagues reported a response to lithium at the end of 6 weeks of acute treatment of only 46.2% (Geller et al 1998). Kowatch et al reported similar response rates in manic children randomized to lithium, carbamazepine or valproate monotherapy (Kowatch et al 2000).

If a patient cannot tolerate a combination of mood stabilizers because of side-effects, then adding a low dose of an atypical antipsychotic agent like risperidone, olanzapine, quetiapine or ziprasidone is another treatment tactic. In an adult BPD study, the authors evaluated the efficacy of olanzapine (5–20 mg/d) versus placebo when added to ongoing mood stabilizer therapy as measured by reductions in Young Mania Rating Scale (YMRS) scores. In this multi-site study, patients with bipolar disorder ($n = 344$), manic or mixed episode, who were inadequately responsive to more than 2 weeks of lithium or valproate therapy, were randomized to receive 'cotherapy' (olanzapine + mood stabilizer) or monotherapy (placebo + mood stabilizer). The study period consisted of a 6 week, acute, double blind phase of co-therapy during which the levels of lithium and valproate were maintained in the therapeutic range. The median duration of monotherapy with a mood stabilizer was 67 days. The authors reported that cotherapy with olanzapine significantly improved patients' YMRS total scores more than monotherapy.

Clinical response rates (50% improvement on YMRS) were significantly higher with cotherapy. Olanzapine cotherapy also improved 21-item Hamilton Depression Rating Scale (HAMD-21) total scores significantly more than monotherapy (4.98 versus 0.89 points). In patients with mixed-episodes with moderate to severe depressive symptoms (DSM-IV mixed episode; HAMD-21 score of 20 at baseline), olanzapine cotherapy improved HAMD-21 scores by 10.31 points compared with 1.57 for monotherapy. Extrapyramidal symptoms were not significantly changed from baseline to end point in either treatment group. Treatment-emergent symptoms that were significantly higher for the olanzapine cotherapy group included somnolence, dry mouth, increased appetite, weight gain, tremor, and slurred speech.

In Chapter 7 it is noted that Delbello and colleagues have also recently demonstrated that quetiapine in combination with divalproex was more effective for the treatment of adolescent bipolar mania than divalproex alone. Treatment with clozapine can be used as a last resort, but is difficult to maintain in the long-term because of the necessity for weekly blood draws for white blood cell counts and the large weight gain and other side-effects often seen with this agent.

## The BPD patient with ADHD

A significant proportion (70–98%) of pediatric bipolar subjects have comorbid ADHD and require additional treatment of the ADHD before they become 'well'. The typical clinical presentation in this scenario is a prepubertal child, who was diagnosed with ADHD at early age and subsequently treated ineffectively with moderate to high doses of stimulants alone around the age of 4–5 years for 'severe irritable hyperactivity'. Then, usually at the age of 7–8 years, the child's bipolar symptoms become very severe with constant mood swings. In the majority of such cases, even after the child's stimulant medications are discontinued, the child continues to manifest severe mood lability and other bipolar symptoms. Once they are started on a mood stabilizer, their mood improves, but they continue to manifest ADHD. Many times, the addition of a low dose stimulant to the mood stabilizer improves the child's ADHD symptoms without exacerbating their mood disorder. These observations are gaining credence among the majority of experts in the field but run against some clinical views that stimulants may exacerbate manic symptoms in bipolar patients (Goodwin and Jamison 1990; DelBello et al 2001). Yet, Carlson et al reported that in a group of seven hospitalized children with bipolar symptoms, the addition of methylphenidate to lithium was beneficial (Carlson et al 1992). Max et al reported an excellent response to dextroamphetamine in a 14-year-old male with an organic bipolar disorder (Max et al 1995). Our clinical experience and the experience of others, suggests that if a pediatric bipolar patient with comorbid ADHD is first stabilized on one or more mood stabilizers, that the addition of a stimulant is often very helpful in treating their comorbid ADHD (Biederman et al 1999). The critical issue appears to be the sequence of treatment, with the patient's bipolar disorder treated with mood stabilizers before low-dose stimulant medication is added or reintroduced.

The overall strategy in this scenario is that once the patient had a positive mood response (rated as 'much' or 'very-much' improved) to a mood stabilizer like valproate or lithium, it helpful to reassess their ADHD symptoms with an ADHD rating scale like the Conner's Teacher and Parent Questionnaire. If they are still manifesting significant ADHD symptoms despite a positive response to the mood stabilizer, then it is often beneficial to start the patient on a low dose of a long-acting stimulant medication. Many times, despite a negative mood response to stimulant monotherapy in the past, the addition of a stimulant to a mood stabilizer is often beneficial for treating the patient's comorbid ADHD without exacerbating their bipolar disorder. Specific tactics include adding a morning dose of long-acting stimulant like Concerta, Adderall XR or Metadate CD.

## The euphoric BPD patient

There is a sub-group of bipolar children and adolescents who present with clear periods of euphoria and who are closer in their BPD phenomenology to adult bipolars. However, these patients are much less common than the complex cycling and irritable manic children discussed above. In these traditional BPD patients, a trial of lithium carbonate may be helpful in many cases, particularly if there are clear periods of euphoria. Specific tactics include obtaining a complete lithium laboratory work-up with an EKG, blood count, urine analysis, BUN, serum creatinine and thyroid functions. The starting does of lithium in outpatients is 25 mg/kg/day in two divided doses. Sustained release preparations like Lithobid and Eskalith are better tolerated in many children than generic lithium carbonate. Children excrete lithium at a higher rate than adults (Vitiello et al 1988) and it is many times necessary to administer the sustained release preparations of lithium twice daily. One problem with lithium is that it sometimes takes 6–8 weeks to get a full response. Due to this long latency for a mood response, it sometimes helpful and necessary to add a low dose of atypical antipsychotic agent until the lithium becomes fully effective. Another tactic for non- or partial-responders is to add another mood stabilizer like valproate or oxcarbazepine to lithium. These agents will often help insomnia and anxiety symtoms.

### The BPD patient with psychosis

Children and adolescents with a psychotic manic or depressive episode many times require treatment with a mood-stabilizing agent and an atypical antipsychotic agent. The strategy in this scenario is to concurrently start both a mood stabilizer and an atypical antipsychotic. Specific tactics include initiating valproate at 20 mg/kg/day in two–three divided doses and olanzapine 2.5–5.0 mg twice daily. Once the manic psychosis has cleared – which may take days to weeks – it may be possible to reduce the patient's atypical antipsychotic dose, while maintaining the mood-stabilizing agent at therapeutic levels. These patients present the greatest risk of relapse and hospitalization when their psychotropic agents are stopped.

### The BPD patient with depression

Many children and adolescents with a BPD may develop depressive symptoms despite treatment with lithium or valproate. The basic strategy for these patients is to maximize the serum levels of whatever mood stabilizer they are on before adding an antidepressant agent. Other specific tactics include adding a low-dose of a serotonin-selective re-uptake inhibitor (SSRI) like citalopram at a dose of 10 mg/day. Other options include bupropion SR or other SSRIs. When combing an SSRI with a mood stabilizer in a child or adolescent with BPD it is important to monitor the patient's mood and behavior carefully for any signs of mania as these agents can sometimes precipitate a manic- or hypo-manic episode. It is conventional wisdom that antidepressants should be tapered while the mood stabilizer is continued, 6–12 weeks after remission of the patient's depressive episode but new data in adults suggest that this may increase the risk of relapse into depression. Adjunctive gabaperitin (Neurotonin®) is widely utilized for persisting insomnia, anxiety and depression in adults but its utility in young children has not been systematically assessed.

## Common issues during treatment

### Duration of treatment

Among adult BPD patients, lithium has been shown to be effective in preventing episodes of mania and episode of depression and in decreasing the rate of suicide (Tondo et al 1998). There is only one study of adolescents with BPD that provides useful guidelines about the duration of treatment. Strober et al followed a group of adolescents who had been hospitalized for a manic episode for five years and demonstrated a three-fold increase in relapse rates among adolescent manics who discontinued lithium after hospital discharge (Strober et al 1990). It is reasonable, based upon this study and studies among adults, to maintain a child or adolescent who has had a single manic episode, on a mood stabilizing agent for 12–18 months. Then, if they are euthymic and asymptomatic, to very gradually reduce the mood stabilizing agent over a 2–3 month period. If BPD symptoms recur the mood-stabilizing agent should be reintroduced and maintained for long term prophylaxis. Ultimately, the benefits of long-term treatment and illness prevention will have to be weighed against the small risks of long-term maintenance treatment and the very large risks of illness exacerbation and progression in the absence of such intervention in any decision made by the patient and their guardians about how long to continue treatment. If a patient has had a manic, mixed or depressive episode that has necessitated hospitalization or has otherwise been incapacitated by the illness, then the benefits of continued treatment with mood stabilizers often outweigh the risks of long-term treatment.

## Insomnia

Many pediatric BPD patients will complain of insomnia. A useful treatment strategy developed by Dr Susan McElroy for adults with BPD is to treat according to the cause of the patient's insomnia. If it is because the patient is still having manic symptoms at the end of the evening that are causing initial insomnia, then it may be helpful to shift whatever mood stabilizers they are taking to an hour before bedtime and insure that these medications are maximized. If the insomnia is caused by anxiety, than adding either gabapentin or a low dose of an atypical antipsychotic agent to whatever mood stabilizer the patient is already taking may be helpful.

## Weight gain

Weight gain is a major side-effect of many mood stabilizers and most atypical antipsychotics. Useful strategies are to stress diet and exercise with restriction of high caloric foods as much as possible. One specific tactic for weight gain is to add a low dose of topiramate to problematic mood stabilizers and or antipsychotic agents. A typical starting dose of topiramate for this problem is 25 mg/day for the first week, 25 mg twice daily for another week and then 50 mg twice daily with further upward titration as necessary to suppress appetite. In the best of both worlds, one might see weight loss as well as better mood stabilization.

## Sedation

The teachers of many pediatric bipolar patients will notice that the child falls asleep in school and that this seriously impairs their learning ability. One strategy for this common problem is to divide the doses of mood stabilizers and atypical antipsychotic agents into two or three smaller doses and give the majority of the sedating medications at bedtime.

## Enuresis

Both nocturnal and daytime enuresis is a common problem when lithium is prescribed particularly in young boys. The first step in these cases is to rule out any medical conditions that might be causing or exacerbating this problem including genital-urinary deformations, renal impairment, or urinary tract infections. A specific tactic is the use of oral DDVAP, 1–2 mg/day. Another tactic is to switch the patient from lithium to valproate or oxcarbamazepine, which do not typically cause enuresis.

## Further reading

Bauer MS, AM Callahan, C Jampala et al (1999) Clinical practice guidelines for bipolar disorder from the Department of Veterans Affairs. *J Clin Psychiatry* **60**: 9–21.

Biederman J, Mick E, Prince J et al (1999) Systematic chart review of the pharmacologic treatment of comorbid attention deficit hyperactivity disorder in youth with bipolar disorder. *J Child Adolesc Psychopharmacol* **9**: 247–56.

Carlson GA, Rapport MD, Kelly KL et al (1992) The effects of methylphenidate and lithium on attention and activity level. *J Am Acad Child Adolesc Psychiatry* **31**: 262–70.

DelBello M, Soutullo C, Hendricks W et al (2001) Prior stimulant treatment in adolescents with bipolar disorder: association with age at onset. *Bipolar Disord* **3**: 53–7.

Frye M, Ketter T, Leverich G et al (2000) The increasing use of polypharmacotherapy for refractory mood disorders: 22 years of study. *J Clin Psychiatry* **61**: 9–15.

Geller B, Cooper TB, Sun K et al (1998) Double-blind and placebo-controlled study of lithium for adolescent bipolar disorders with secondary substance dependency. *J Am Acad Child Adolesc Psychiatry* **37**: 171–78.

Geller B, Sun K, Zimerman B et al (1995) Complex and rapid-cycling in bipolar children and adoescents: a preliminary study. *J Affect Disord* **34**: 259–68.

Geller B, Zimerman B, Williams M et al (2000) Diagnostic characteristics of 93 cases of a prepubertal and early adolescent bipolar disorder phenotype by gender, puberty and comorbid attention deficit hyperactivity disorder. *J Child Adolesc Pyschopharmacology* **10**: 157–64.

Goldberg JF (2000) Treatment guidelines: current and future management of bipolar disorder. *J Clin Psych* **61 (Suppl 13)**: 12–8.

Goodwin FK, Jamison KR (1990) *Manic–Depressive Illness*. New York: Oxford University Press.

Grof P, Alda M, Grof E et al (1994) Lithium response and genetics of affective disorders. *J Affect Disord* **32**: 85–95.

Kovacs M, Pollock M (1995) Bipolar disorder and comorbid conduct disorder in childhood and adolescence. *J Am Acad Child Adolesc Psychiatry* **34**: 715–23.

Kowatch RA, Suppes T, Carmody TJ et al (2000) Effect size of lithium, divalproex sodium, and carbamazepine in children and adolescents with bipolar disorder. *J Am Acad Child Adolesc Psychiatry* **39**: 713–20.

Max JE, Richards L, Hamdan-Allen G (1995) Case study: antimanic effectiveness of dextroamphetamine in a brain-injured adolescent. *J Am Acad Child Adolesc Psychiatry* **34**: 472–6.

McClellan J, Werry JS (1997) Practice parameters for the assessment and treatment of children and adolescents with bipolar disorder. *J Am Acad Child Adolesc Psychiatry* **36**(suppl): 157S–176S.

Post RM (1993) Issues in the long-term management of bipolar affective illness. *Psychiatric Annals* **23**: 86–93.

Prien RF, Rush AJ (1996) National Institute of Mental Health Workshop Report on the Treatment of Bipolar Disorder. *Biol Psychiatry* **40**: 215–20.

Rush A (1999) Strategies and tactics in the management of maintenance treatment for depressed patients. *J Clin Psychiatry* **60**(suppl 14): 21–6.

Sachs G, Printz D, Kahn D et al (2000) The Expert Consensus Guideline Series: Medication Treatment of Bipolar Disorder 2000. *Postgraduate Medicine* **Spec No**(Apr): 1–104.

Solomon DA, Keitner GI, Ryan CE et al (1996) Polypharmacy in bipolar I disorder. *Psychopharmacol Bull* **32**: 579–87.

Strober M, Morrell W, Lampert C et al (1990) Relapse following discontinuation of lithium maintenance therapy in adolescents with bipolar I illness: a naturalistic study. *Am J Psychiatry* **147**: 457–61.

Suppes T, Rush AJJ, Kraemer AC et al (1998). Treatment algorithm use to optimize management of symptomatic patients with a history of mania. *J Clin Psychiatry* **59**: 89–96; quiz 97–8.

Tondo L, Baldessarini RJ, Hennen J et al (1998). Lithium treatment and risk of suicidal behavior in bipolar disorder patients. *J Clin Psychiatry* **59**: 405–14.

Vitiello B, Behar D, Malone R et al (1988). Pharmacokinetics of lithium carbonate in children. *J Clin Psychopharmacol* **8**: 355–9.

West SA, McElroy SL, Strakowski SM et al (1995). Attention deficit hyperactivity disorder in adolescent mania. *Am J Psychiatry* **152**: 271–3.

Wozniak J, Biederman J, Kiely K et al (1995). Mania-like symptoms suggestive of childhood-onset bipolar disorder in clinically referred children. *J Am Acad Child Adolesc Psychiatry* **34**: 867–76.

# chapter 10

# Therapeutic and educational issues

## Therapeutic issues

Children and adolescents with a bipolar disorder have an evolving, biological illness that interacts with the familial, psychosocial, and educational environment in which they are rapidly developing. In the last several chapters we have emphasized psychopharmacology as the mainstay of treatment because there is a strong biological component to pediatric bipolar disorders. However, it is also important to understand that the development of a strong treatment alliance with these patients and their families is critical to successful treatment of pediatric bipolar disorder (BPD). Many years ago, when one of us was a resident in training, we complained one day to our supervisor about an adult patient with a bipolar disorder who had stopped taking his lithium shortly after hospital discharge and was subsequently re-hospitalized with another manic episode. This sage supervisor, replied, 'Robert, this patient will take his lithium when he trusts you.'. This advice is important to keep in mind when working with patients and families who struggle with a child or adolescent with BPD. These families are often frustrated because of a lack of accurate diagnosis and ineffective treatments, and are desperate to find a psychiatrist who understands the complexity of pediatric bipolar disorders and who demonstrates that they can be relied upon and trusted.

There are numerous psychosocial, educational and therapeutic issues that arise when treating a child or adolescent with a BPD. In this chapter we will provide strategies that a treating psychiatrist can use in combination with pharmaco-therapy with these patients. In children and adolescents with BPD, no specific form of psychotherapy has been shown to be superior to another. However, it is important that the child or adolescent with BPD be involved with a therapist who is familiar with this disorder and who understands the difficulties that these patients experience. This therapist could be the treating psychiatrist or another therapist who is willing to collaborate with the psychiatrist about the patient. The model we have found to be the most useful is a chronic illness model, similar to those used in the management of asthma or diabetes in children and adolescents. In this model, education about the illness and medication compliance is emphasized.

Many of these patients are at increased risk for the several high-risk behaviors and it is helpful to anticipate these issues and begin discussing them with pediatric BPD patients and their families before they arise. These include:

## Substance abuse

Substance abuse is a significant problem in adolescents with BPD. West and colleagues reported that 40% of adolescent inpatients with BPD met criteria for substance use disorders (West et al 1996). Wilens and colleagues at Harvard found adolescents with adolescent-onset BPD were nine times more likely to abuse various substances like marijuana and alcohol, than those adolescents with childhood-onset BPD. This suggests that patients who develop BPD during adolescence are particularly prone to substance use and abuse (Wilens et al 1999). Our clinical experience is that 50–70% of bipolar adolescents will use, and sometimes abuse, various substances including alcohol, marijuana, ecstasy, amphetamines and various hallucinogens. The rate of substance use among normal adolescents is estimated to between 40–54% (US Department of Health and Human Services 2001), so the rate among bipolar adolescents is higher than among adolescents without BPD.

This increased rate of substance use in adolescents with BPD appears to be due to a combination of factors including BPD patient's frequent attempts at self-medication of anxiety, depression and ADHD, increased adolescent risk-taking, and manic grandiosity – 'I'm special and cannot get addicted to drugs.' Adolescents with BPD should be counseled that most substances will ultimately, if not initially, make the symptoms of their mood disorder worse and should be avoided or at best minimized. Hallucinogens should be avoided totally as they will often precipitate a psychotic manic episode from which it is difficult to recover. Caffeine should also be minimized as too many double-lattes can cause insomnia and sleep loss which can precipitate or exacerbate a manic episode.

## Sexuality

Many normal adolescents are sexually active but adolescents with BPD can become 'hypersexual' during a manic episode. The hypersexual behavior during a manic episode is qualitatively different than the sexual behavior of a child or adolescent with PTSD. In a manic child or adolescent their sexual behavior is often erotic and pleasure seeking as compared to the child or adolescent with PTSD, where this behavior is anxiety driven and more compulsive in nature. It is important to discuss the risk of impulsive and manic-driven sexual behavior with BPD adolescents and their parents before it occurs. The risks of excessive involvement with erotic materials on the Internet and other sources should also be discussed with the patient. The dangers of sexually transmitted diseases and possible adverse effects of psychotropic medications on a fetus should also be discussed with female BPD adolescents and their parents. A plan for a reliable birth control should be implemented in consultation with the patient's pediatrician or gynecologist. Sexually active BPD females can be started on the newer, low progestogene birth-control pills that are less likely to effect their mood or interact with whatever psychotropic agents they are on. It may be prudent for women of child-bearing age to be on folate (1 mg/day at a minimum) 'just in case'. Folate 5–10 mg/day can likely help prevent spontaneous and drug-related birth defects and may also potentiate antidepressant effects.

## Suicide

Adults, adolescents and children with BPD are at greatly increased risk for suicide attempts and completions. Data from the Epidemiologic Catchment Area study revealed that the lifetime rates of suicide attempts of adults with BPD was 29.2% (Chen and Dilsaver 1996). In the largest and most well-designed population study of adolescents with bipolar disorders to date, Lewinsohn and colleagues reported that 44% of adolescents with a bipolar disorder had been suicidal at some time during a one-year period of assessment (Lewinsohn et al 1995). Geller and colleagues reported that in a sample of 93 outpatients with BPD, and a mean age of 11 years, that 23% were suicidal (Geller et al 2000). Suicidal ideation and attempts should be taken very seriously in these patients and require active intervention with the patient and their family.

## Peer relations

Peer relations can be very difficult for these patients due to their frequent mood swings, poor social skills, and impulsive behaviors. This is a major issue that can be worked with in therapy to develop more appropriate social skills. Sometimes referral to a social skills group is also helpful. These patients should be encouraged to participate in as many outside activities as their schedule reasonably allows, but should be counseled to limit excessive activities and over commitments so as to not cause further stressors that may exacerbate their BPD.

## Siblings

The siblings of these patients often get overlooked in the tumult surrounding the BPD child or adolescent's illness. These youngsters often feel neglected, overwhelmed, and afraid to voice their feelings because of the amount of family time and energy already devoted to the sibling with BPD. It is important to include these individuals in discussions about the effects that their sibling's BPD illness is having upon themselves and the family and to intervene with special patient support and attention when necessary.

## Medication compliance

The majority of available evidence about the various psychotropic agents used to treat children and adolescents with BPD suggests that they can be effective if taken on a regular basis. However, compliance is a major problem for patients with pediatric and especially adolescent BPD. It is very difficult for a BPD child or adolescent to take two to three medications, two to three times a day, every day, for a prolonged and often unspecified period of time. The risks of medication noncompliance include negative psychosocial effects, rehospitalization and potential suicide. The only study about the effects of medication compliance and non-compliance on outcome in adolescents with BPD, was by Strober et al who reported a threefold increase in relapse rates among adolescent with BPD who discontinued lithium after hospital discharge compared with those who remained on lithium (Strober et al 1990).

The risks of medication noncompliance should be discussed with the patient and their family on an ongoing basis. Patients and their families should be educated about the common and potential adverse effects of the psychotropic medications that they are prescribed and any concerns addressed before the medication is started. An excellent resource for patients and parents about the adverse effects of psychotropic medication is the book, *Helping Parents, Youth, and Teachers Understand Medications for Behavioral and Emotional Problems: A Resource Book of Medication Information Handouts* by Dulcan and Benton (Dulcan and Benton 2002). Basco and Rush's book on cognitive and behavioral approach to compliance is filled with good ideas and strategies. Long acting medications and medications that are better tolerated should be used whenever possible to enhance compliance as should HS or BID dosing whenever possible.

## Mood charting

A useful tool for patients, families and clinicians is prospective mood chart using the Kiddie Life Chart Method (LCM) developed by Gabriel Leverich and Robert Post, of NIMH. These charts are simply a scaled calendar on which the parent or the patient can indicate if they were more 'activated' or 'withdrawn' on a daily basis. Prospective mood charting with a chart like the LCM allows that patient and their parents to objectively chart and monitor their mood cycling. This is useful in two ways – this allows the patient and their parents to see that there is a mood disorder present and that they are not simply a 'bad kid' or 'bad' parents and it is very quick way of summarizing the pattern and severity of a patient's past and current mood states. These charts can be reviewed by the clinician at each visit and changes in medication made accordingly. Most parents and patients find these charts very useful, whereas others do not have the time or insight necessary to complete them. A blank copy of the Kiddie LCM chart is illustrated in Figure 10.1.

## Educational issues

Children and adolescents with BPD often have difficulty in school because of their frequent and severe mood swings, the medications they are required to take that many times are sedating, and comorbid learning disabilities. Wozniak et al reported that in a clinically referred sample of 43 children with BPD, 30% had an arithmetic learning disability, 42% had a reading disability and 33% were placed in a special class (Wozniak et al 1995).

The rights of a BPD child or adolescent with disabilities to a free and appropriate education are protected by several federal laws. The most important US law is the Individuals with Disabilities Education Act of 1997 (IDEA) (US Department of Education 2001). Under IDEA, a child is guaranteed a free and appropriate education in the 'least restrictive environment' along with all appropriate 'related services' required to enable a child to benefit from his or her education. According to IDEA children aged between 3 and 21, who need special education and related services because of a disabling condition, are eligible. A child with a disability is defined as one with mental retardation; a hearing impairment or deafness; a speech or language impairment; a visual impairment, including blindness; emotional disturbance; an orthopedic impairment;

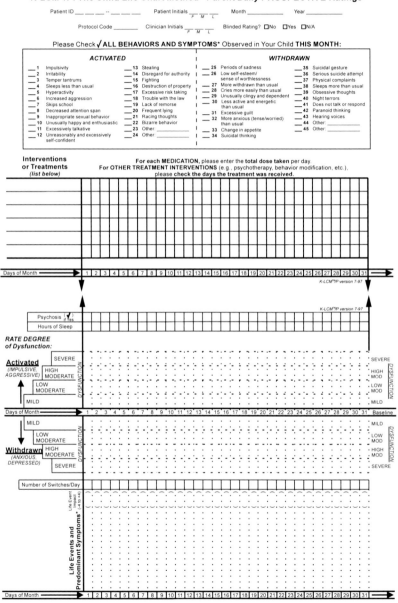

**Figure 10.1** *Reproduced with permission from Leverick GS, Post RM (1998) Life charting of affective disorders.* CNS Spectrums 3: 21–37.

autism; traumatic brain injury; another health impairment; a specific learning disability; deaf-blindness or multiple disabilities. Most BPD children will qualify because of the emotional problems that their BPD causes and or their comorbid ADHD.

There are three issues to identify when attempting to help a BPD child or adolescent in their educational system:

(i) Are their educational needs being met in their current school environment?

(ii) Besides the child's bipolar disorder, are their other disorders, particularly ADHD or learning disabilities, that need to be remediated?

(iii) What resources do the parents of the child need to effectively insure that their child's educational needs are met in their school system?

As discussed above, many children and adolescents will have comorbid ADHD and or learning disabilities that require additional medication and resources. Table 10.1 contains general guidelines for screening for a learning disability (LD). If a LD is suspected, the patient should be referred for educational testing. This is best done when the child is not

Table 10.1 Possible signs of a learning disability once mood is adequately stabilized

- Trouble with understanding written assignments and other readings.
- Specific problems in mathematics, science, and/or foreign languages.
- Trouble with completing written assignments (production of information, spelling, grammar).
- Trouble keeping up with reading assignments or remembering what was read.
- Not having enough time to complete examinations or trouble with specific types of tests (i.e. multiple-choice, essay).
- Receiving poorer than expected grades for IQ.
- Feeling constantly overwhelmed and demoralized with the academic workload.

in a major affective episode and is relatively stabilized on medications. Otherwise manic inattention or depressive cognitive impairment will obscure the results and interpretation. Often, an educational consultant can help guide parents through the IEP process. Another useful resource for parents is, *The Complete IEP Guide: How to Advocate for Your Special Ed Child* by Lawrence M Siegel.

The goal of treatment with these patients is to allow them to function as normally as possible within their families, schools and peer groups. Their success in life will be determined by the successful stabilization of their mood, remediation of any learning disabilities including ADHD, and development of appropriate social skills and peer relationships. This is a challenge for the patient, their family, and treating clinicians, but can be accomplished with ongoing attention to finding and optimizing the appropriate treatments.

## Further reading

Chen YW, Dilsaver SC (1996) Lifetime rates of suicide attempts among subjects with bipolar and unipolar disorders relative to subjects with other axis I disorders. *Biol Psychiatry* **39**: 896–9.

Dulcan M, Benton T (2002) *Helping Parents, Youth, And Teachers Understand Medications For Behavioral And Emotional Problems: A Resource Book Of Medication Information Handouts* 2nd Ed. Washington DC: American Psychiatric Press.

Geller B, Zimerman B, Williams M et al (2000) Diagnostic characteristics of 93 cases of a prepubertal and early adolescent bipolar disorder phenotype by gender, puberty and comorbid attention deficit hyperactivity disorder. *J Child Adolesc Pychopharmacol* **10**: 157–64.

Lewinsohn PM, Klein DN, Seeley JR (1995) Bipolar disorders in a community sample of older adolescents: prevalence, phenomenology, comorbidity, and course. *J Am Acad Child Adolesc Psychiatry* **34**: 454–63.

Strober M, Morrell W, Lampert C (1990) Relapse following discontinuation of lithium maintenance therapy in adolescents with bipolar I illness: A naturalistic study. *Am J Psychiatry* **147**: 457–61.

US Department of Education (2001) The Individuals With Disabilities Education Act Amendments of 1997.

US Department of Health And Human Services (2001) Monitoring The Future: National Results On Adolescent Drug Use, US Department Of Health/NIH.

West SA, Strakowski SM, Sax KW et al (1996) Phenomenology and comorbidity of adolescents hospitalized for the treatment of acute mania. *Biol Psychiatry* **39**: 458–60.

Wilens TE, Biederman J, Millstein RB et al (1999) Risk for substance use disorders in youths with child- and adolescent-onset bipolar disorder. *J Am Acad Child Adolesc Psychiatry* **38**: 680–5.

Wozniak J, Biederman J, KielyK et al (1995) Mania-like symptoms suggestive of childhood-onset bipolar disorder in clinically referred children. *J Am Acad Child Adolesc Psychiatry* **34**: 867–76.

# chapter 11

# Conclusions

– Ask not what disease the person has, but rather what person the
disease has.

(attributed to) William Osler

Over the last ten years the field of pediatric bipolar illness has been
developing rapidly. It is now recognized that pediatric bipolar disorders
are prevalent (Lewinsohn et al 1995) and that they often seriously
disrupt the lives of children, adolescents and their families. Recent
studies show that patients with bipolar disorders (BPD) have poorer academic performance, disturbed interpersonal relationships, increased
rates of substance abuse, legal difficulties, multiple hospitalizations, and
increased rates of both suicide attempts and completions (Akiskal et al
1985; Lewinsohn et al 1995; Strober et al 1995; Lewinsohn et al 2000;
Nottelmann 2001).

There is emerging evidence that the phenomenology of pediatric BPD
disorders is frequently different than adults with BPD. Pediatric patients
often present with a mixed or 'dysphoric' picture characterized by frequent short periods of intense mood liability and irritability rather than
classic euphoric mania. Geller and colleagues reported that in 93 bipolar
children and adolescents that, 'complex' cycling patterns occurred, char-

acterized by brief manic periods lasting four or more hours, occurred in 77.4% of these subjects (Geller et al 2000). Perhaps, DSM-V will recognize the data from recent studies and include diagnostic criteria for pediatric bipolar disorders that are developmentally appropriate. It is often difficult to fit the 'round peg' of pediatric bipolarity into the 'square hole' of current adult DSM-IV bipolar criteria and the category of BP-NOS (not otherwise specified should be utilized accordingly).

During the 1970s and 1980s the majority of substantive work in pediatric bipolar disorders was done by Gabriele Carlson at Stony Brook, State University of New York (Carlson 1978, 1984; Carlson and Kashani 1988), Michael Strober at UCLA (Strober and Carlson 1982; Strober et al 1988) and Elizabeth Weller at Ohio State University (Weller et al 1986; Weller et al 1987). In the last ten years the lion's share of research in pediatric bipolar disorders has been done at two centers: the Harvard group led by Joseph Biederman with Janet Wozniak, Tim Wilens and Jean Frazier; and the Washington University team led by Barbara Geller. Both of these groups have published many significant, evidence-based studies in the last several years despite academic controversy generating resistance to the publication of their data. Their studies showed that pediatric bipolar disorders do exist, often present differently than adult bipolar disorders, and can be treated with mood stabilizers and other psychotropic agents widely used in adults.

There are several exciting areas of research emerging from other investigators in the field. Kiki Chang at Stanford is studying children of bipolar parents who present with various behavioral problems but do not yet meet criteria for a bipolar disorder I or II. Chang is finding that treatment with valproate is effective in treating these patient's early mood and behavioral problems with the hope being that these early interventions will prevent the emergence of the full BPD picture. Pablo Davanzo at UCLA is using magnetic resonance spectroscopy to explore the neurobiology of pediatric biology disorders and to predict response to lithium. The Harvard group with Biederman, Wozniak, Frazier and Wilens is continuing their pioneering work with innovative pharmacological treatments for pediatric BPD. Boris Birmaher at the Western Psychiatric Institute and Clinic in Pittsburgh is conducting a longitudinal study of bipolar children to determine the range of long-term outcomes. Melissa DelBello recently published the first controlled study that showed the combination of the atypical agent quetiapine with valproate was significantly more effective than valproate alone. She is now directly comparing pediatric BPD patients treated with valproate versus those treated with quetiapine (DelBello et al 2002). Barbara Geller continues her longitudinal studies about the phenomenology and course of PBD. Her studies are defining the clinical characteristics and course of these patients – something that is critical to this field.

The challenges to this field include:

- The development and testing of medications that are truly effective mood stabilizers (i.e. treat all phases of this illness without exacerbating either the manic or depressed phases) and are safe and well-tolerated in children.
- The development of pharmaco-genetic assays for the better prediction of individual treatment response.
- Finding genetic probes for early diagnosis and sub typing.
- Conducting neuroimaging studies that reveal pathophysiology and aid in the prediction of treatment response.
- The development of effective cognitive and behavioral therapies specifically for children with bipolar illness disorders and which can augment pharmacotherapy.
- Exploring and revealing of the basic neurobiology of this disorder in the hope of more completely treating and ultimately preventing it from developing.

In 1960 two child psychoanalysts wrote that 'The authors believe that the occurrence of manic-depression in early childhood as a clinical phenomenon has yet to be demonstrated' (Anthony and Scott 1960). Fortunately for the field at about this same time, a pediatric neurologist, Warren Weinberg, was seeing many children with severe mood swings and other manic behaviors, in the pediatric neurology clinic at Washington University. Weinberg, by virtue of his training in neurology, was not blinded by psychiatric dogma and was able to recognize this phenomenon for what it was – the early expression of bipolar disorders that was similar to, but different from the adult bipolar phenotype.

What the field of pediatric bipolarity desperately needs now are more systematic, controlled and comparative studies about effective treatments for these disorders that are informed, but not encumbered, by adult BPD research. In the future we look forward to: studies about the use of 'rational combination pharmacotherapy' as the majority of these patients do not respond to treatment with a single mood stabilizer; the development of specific cognitive-behavioral therapies for this disorder; and the increased use of emerging technologies in genetics, molecular biology, and neuro-imaging to aid clinicians in diagnosis and treatment. We owe this to our pediatric patients with bipolar illness and their families.

## Further reading

Akiskal HS, Downs J, Jordan P et al (1985) Affective disorders in referred children and younger siblings of manic-depressives. Mode of onset and prospective course. *Arch Gen Psychiatry* **42**(10): 996–1003.

Anthony J, Scott P (1960) Manic-depressive psychosis in childhood. *Child Psychol Psychiatry* **4**: 53–72.

Carlson GA (1984) Classification issues of bipolar disorders in childhood. *Psychiatric Dev* **2**(4): 273–85.

Carlson GA, Kashani JH (1988) Manic symptoms in a non-referred adolescent population. *J Affect Disorder* **15**(3): 219–26.

Carlson S (1978) Manic-depressive illness in early adolescence: clinical and diagnostic characteristics in six cases. *J Am Acad Child Adolesc Psychiatry* **17**: 138–53.

Delbello M, Schwiers M, Rosenberg H et al (2002) Quetiapine as adjunctive treatment for adolescent mania associated with bipolar disorder. *J Am Acad Child Adolesc Psychiatry* (in press).

Geller B, Zimerman B, Williams M et al (2000) Diagnostic characteristics of 93 cases of a prepubertal and early adolescent bipolar disorder phenotype by gender, puberty and comorbid attention deficit hyperactivity disorder. *J Child Adolesc Psychopharmacol* **10**: 157–64.

Lewinsohn P, Klein D, Seeley J (2000) Bipolar disorder during adolescence and young adulthood in a community sample. *Bipolar Disord* **2**(3 Pt 2): 281–93.

Lewinsohn PM, Klein DN, Seeley JR (1995) Bipolar disorders in a community sample of older adolescents: prevalence, phenomenology, comorbidity, and course. *J Am Acad Child Adolesc Psychiatry* **34**: 454–63.

Nottelmann E (2001) National institute of mental health research roundtable on prepubertal bipolar disorder. *J Am Acad Child Adolesc Psychiatry* **40**(August): 871–78.

Strober M, Carlson G (1982) Bipolar illness in adolescents with major depression: clinical, genetic, and psychopharmacologic predictors in a three- to four-year prospective follow-up investigation. *Arch Gen Psychiatry* **39**(5): 549–55.

Strober M, Morrell M, Burroughs J et al (1988. A family study of bipolar I disorder in adolescence. Early onset of symptoms linked to increased familial loading and lithium resistance. *J Affect Disord* **15**(3): 255–68.

Strober M, Schmidt-Lackner S, Freeman R et al (1995) Recovery and relapse in adolescents with bipolar affective illness: a five-year naturalistic, prospective follow-up. *J Am Acad Child Adolesc Psychiatry* **34**(6): 724–31.

Weller EB, Weller RA, Fristad MA (1986) Lithium dosage guide for prepubertal children: a preliminary report. *J Am Acad Child Psychiatry* **25**(1): 92–5.

Weller EB, Weller RA, Fristad MA et al (1987) Saliva lithium monitoring in prepubertal children. *J Am Acad Child Adolesc Psychiatry* **26**(2): 173–5.

# chapter 12

# Resources for clinicians

There are an increasing number of text and online resources available to the clinician about pediatric bipolar disorders. Many of these resources are extremely useful for families and patients with bipolar disorder (BPD). Below are summarized the resources that we have found to be the most useful when working with these children and their families.

## Print materials

A recent search of Amazon.com found 64 books about bipolar disorders. The books that we have found the most useful for working with these children and their families were:

**The Bipolar Child: The Definitive and Reassuring Guide to Childhood's Most Misunderstood Disorder** by Demitri Papolos, MD and Janice Papolos (Broadway Books, revised edition due in September 2002).

This was the first book written expressly about pediatric BPD for parents and it contains much valuable information for parents about this disorder in children and adolescents.

**Child and Early Adolescent Bipolar Disorder: Theory, Assessment, and Treatment** edited by Geller B, DelBello MP (Guilford Publications 2002).
This is the best academic text about pediatric bipolar disorders. It is the 'Goodwin and Jamison' of pediatric bipolarity.

**Surviving Manic Depression: A Manual on Bipolar Disorder for Patients, Families and Providers** by E Fuller Torrey, MD and Michael B Knable, DO (2002).
This book contains an excellent overview of diagnostic, treatment, and family issues with BPD. It also includes a section on child and adolescent BPD, and extensive information about the various psychotropic medications used to treat this disorder.

**Bipolar Disorders: A Guide to Helping Children & Adolescents** by Mitzi Waltz (O'Reilly, 2000).
This book contains many chapters useful to parents with the last three chapters discussing insurance, school, and transition to adulthood. This book is particularly helpful to families of adolescents with BPD.

**Everything you Need to Know about Bipolar Disorder and Manic Depressive Illness** by Michael A Sommers (Rosen Publishing Group, 2000).
The author offers practical advice to patients for getting the most out of the various treatments that are now available for adults with BPD including medication, psychotherapy, electroconvulsive therapy and transcranial magnetic stimulation. The author also describes problems that are unique to women, the forms the illness takes in children and adolescents, the genetics of the disease, and ways to cope with the stigma of psychiatric diagnosis.

This book is very clear, with examples and a glossary of terms at the back. It is an excellent book for bright and curious adolescents who have just been diagnosed with BPD.

**Bipolar Disorder: A Family-Focused Treatment Approach** by David J Miklowitz and Michael J Goldstein (Guilford Publications Inc., 1997).

This book is written for therapists and contains a psychoeducational family treatment that educates the patient and the family as to the disorder, gives the family ways of coping with the disorder and hospitalization, works on medicinal compliance, and prepares the client and the family for any future episodes. Included is a nine-month outpatient program designed to help adult patients and families understand and manage the effects of bipolar disorder. Families learn about: 1) how to deal with their feelings that their loved one has a serious mental illness, 2) the nature of bipolar disorder, 3) problem solving techniques for difficult situations, 4) how to deal with manic relapses, 5) how to deal with depressive relapses, 6) what to do when you suspect your bipolar family member of substance abuse, and 7) the suicidal crisis.

**Cognitive-Behavioral Therapy for Bipolar Disorder** by Monica Basco, PhD and A John Rush, MD (Guilford Press, 1996).
This book is aimed at therapists who work with adults with BPD, but is useful for understanding how bipolar patients can be helped by identifying and changing negative thinking patterns. This title includes many examples from actual cases. The authors are on faculty at University of Texas Southwestern Medical Center.

**Straight Talk about Psychiatric Medications for Kids** by Timothy E Wilens, MD (The Guilford Press, 1999).
This is an excellent overview of common childhood psychiatric disorders (including bipolar disorder) and medications used to treat them. Dr Wilens is a psychopharmacologist with extensive experience in evaluating and treating pediatric bipolar disorders. This book was recently updated with more information about the use of atypicals and dosing, as well as covering issues of psychiatric comorbidity.

**Helping Parents, Youth, and Teachers Understand Medications for Behavioral and Emotional Problems: A Resource Book of Medication Information Handouts**, 2nd edition by Mina Dulcan, Tami Benton (Editors) (American Psychiatric Press, 2002).
This recently updated book contains handouts providing clear information

about psychiatric medications for children and adolescents, how long they should be taken, what happens if they are suddenly stopped, side effects, and adverse effects, with separate handouts for parents, youth, and teachers. A CD-ROM is also included that contains printable copies of these handouts for patients, parents and teachers.

**It's Nobody's Fault: Getting the Right Help for Your Troubled Child**
by Harold S Koplewicz (Times Books, 1996).
The author covers the major psychiatric disorders in children including BPD and suggests means – including therapy and medication – by which families may lessen the difficulties posed by those disorders. The author offers a great deal of scientific information in a format accessible to parents, and friends of children with psychiatric disorders.

# World Wide Web resources

A search in June 2002 of the World Wide Web using the search engine Google with the term, 'pediatric bipolar disorder' revealed over 14,000 hits. Here are some of the sites that we found particularly useful:

**Child and Adolescent Bipolar Foundation (CABF)** (www.cabf.org)
The Child and Adolescent Bipolar Foundation is a parent-led, non-profit, web-based membership organization of families raising children diagnosed with, or at risk for, early-onset bipolar disorder. The CABF website is an outstanding source of information about this disorder for patients, parents and clinicians. This site also contains a searchable directory of bipolar support groups for families (http://www.cabf.org/community/supportgroups/local/search.asp).

**National Alliance for the Mentally Ill (NAMI)** (www.nami.org)
This website has several pages with good information about child and adolescent BPD, see (http://www.nami.org/helpline/bipolar-child.html). NAMI is one of the best advocacy organizations in the US for people with mental illnesses and their families.

**National Depressive and Manic-Depressive Association (National DMDA)** (http://www.ndmda.org/)

The National Depressive and Manic-Depressive Association (National DMDA) is the nation's largest patient-directed, illness-specific organization. Their mission is to educate patients, families, professionals and the public concerning the nature of depressive and manic-depressive illnesses as *treatable* medical diseases; to foster self-help for patients and families; to eliminate discrimination and stigma; to improve access to care; and to advocate for research toward the elimination of these illnesses.

**National Institute of Mental Health** (http://www.nimh.nih.gov/publicat/childmenu.cfm*)* This website by NIMH offers a list of recent publications regarding children and adolescents with psychiatric disorders. This site includes CRISP (Computer Retrieval of Information on Scientific Projects) (https://www-commons.cit.nih.gov/crisp/) which is a searchable database of federally funded biomedical research projects conducted at universities, hospitals, and other research institutions. Anyone can use the CRISP interface to search for scientific concepts, emerging trends and techniques, or identify specific projects and/or investigators.

**Stanley Foundation Bipolar Network** (http://www.bipolarnetwork. org/)

This website describes multi-center research efforts in BPD by some of the most respected mental health researchers in the US and Europe. The mission of the Bipolar Network is to advance scientific understanding of the causes of bipolar illness and to establish strategies for the best long-term treatment of this illness.

**Federation of Families for Children's Mental Health** (http:// www.ffcmh.org/Eng_one.html)

The Federation of Families for Children's Mental Health is a National parent-run non-profit organization focused on the needs of children and youth with emotional, behavioral or mental disorders and their families. The Federation provides an opportunity for family members to work with professionals and other interested citizens to improve services for their children with emotional, behavioral or mental disorders.

**American Academy of Child and Adolescent Psychiatry Facts for Families** (http://www.aacap.org/publications/factsfam/index.htm)
Norman Alessi of the University of Michigan originally developed AACAP's website and the Facts for Families section has proven to the most popular and useful part of this website. These 'Facts for Families' provide concise and up-to-date information on issues that affect children, adolescents, and their families. These pages may be downloaded from AACAP's website, duplicated and distributed free of charge to parents and others as long as the American Academy of Child and Adolescent Psychiatry is properly credited and no profit is gained from their use.

**Juvenile Bipolar Research Foundation** (www.bpchildresearch.org/index.html)
This site was recently organized by Demitri Papolos, past chair of the CABF Professional Advisory Council and is dedicated to determining the etiology of pediatric bipolar disorders.

Despite the amount of new information about pediatric BPD that is available, this disorder is still frequently misdiagnosed and inadequately treated. The more that patients, families, and clinicians know about the diagnosis, treatment and management of this disorder, the better the short- and long-term outcomes of these patient.

# Index

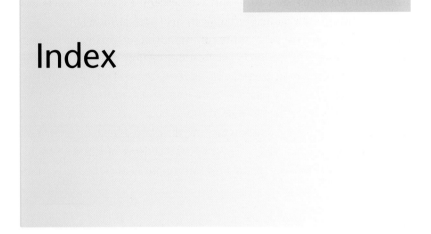

Page numbers in *italic* denote figure legends where there is no textual reference on the same page. BP = bipolar disorder.